CONQUERING
P A I N

An Illustrated Guide to Pain Relief
and Pain Management

Jay B. Forrest, M.D.

1994
Empowering Press
Hamilton, Canada

Distribution

Conquering Pain is distributed in the United States by
Login Publishers Consortium, 1436 W. Randolph, Chicago, IL 60607
and in Canada by General Publishing, 30 Lesmill Road, Don Mills, Ontario M3B 2T6

Information on *Conquering Pain* and other books in this series can be obtained by writing to
Empowering Press, One James Street South, P.O. Box 620, LCD 1, Hamilton, Ontario Canada L8N 3K7

To my wife, Janette.

Acknowledgments

I thank Joanne Taylor for her expert assistance, Leah Aurini for her superb illustrations, and my friend Douglas Tod for his critique.

NOTICE

The authors and publisher have done all they can to make sure that the care recommended in this book reflects the best current practices and standards (this includes choice of medication and dosage). Research, regulations, and clinical practices are constantly changing, so you are encouraged to check all product information sheets from all medication packages. If in doubt about anything in this book or on the product information sheets, contact your personal physician for advice on the proper procedure.

Printed in Canada

ISBN 0-9697781-0-4

CONQUERING   PAIN

Contents

INTRODUCTION

During the past twenty-five years I have treated many thousands of patients who were referred to my clinic because of pain. The great majority had already seen numerous doctors, chiropractors, holistic healers, or acupuncturists, and many had been subjected to multiple surgical procedures without relief of their problems. The most common reasons established medicine has failed these patients are a widespread lack of knowledge about pain and a reluctance to use available and effective remedies. Here you will learn about pain and how it can be conquered. Today, powerful drugs are available for the relief of pain after surgery or injuries, or from disease such as cancer, and new techniques have been introduced for improved control of pain. For the first time in my career as an *algologist* (pain specialist) doctors are showing an increasing awareness of and interest in the treatment of pain as a high priority. As recently as ten years ago, pain management was still unfashionable and doctors who specialized in this area were viewed as a little eccentric. Not so now. Pain clinics and organized acute pain services are increasingly available and soon will be a part of every medium-sized hospital in the Western world. The main reason for this change is that society in general and patients in particular now expect to have more say in matters of health.

There are three things to remember about pain and how we treat it.

1. **Pain is a necessary and unpleasant condition of life.**
The first cry of a newborn child is a response to the sudden impact of unpleasant sensations. The strangeness of its new existence outside the warm, silent, and protected environment of the womb (uterus) causes a rapid arousal of the infant's nervous system. Each of us has seen how a baby's responses become

patterned within a few days after birth as pleasant (baby gurgles, smiles, or sleeps) or unpleasant (baby cries, squirms, holds its little fists tight, and shakes its arms). Hunger is one example of an unpleasant sensation. We talk as adults of having "hunger pains" and our behavior becomes directed towards seeking food to relieve this unpleasant sensation. Pain changes our behavior and our priorities because it disrupts our normal activities as we become more and more preoccupied with finding relief.

The distinguishing feature of all pains is that they are always unpleasant. The International Association for the Study of Pain (IASP) defines pain as "*an unpleasant sensory and emotional experience associated with actual or potential tissue damage or described in terms of such damage*". The important thing about this definition is that it highlights the fact that all pains involve unpleasant bodily sensations and emotional feelings and that the experience of pain is due to some damaging (noxious) change in the tissues of the body.

2. All pains have causes.

The most common cause of pain is damage to tissues from injury or disease. Sometimes pain can exist without any obvious external cause, for example, some types of headache. But there is always a reason for pain even though we may not fully understand what it is. Spontaneous pains or imagined pains simply do not exist. Quite often when a patient is referred to the pain management clinic the doctor's letter says something like, "No physical findings, not coping, functional pain, please help". This can be interpreted as, "I don't know what is wrong with this patient. I've done the usual tests and they are normal so there can't be anything too serious but he's really difficult to deal with". Labelling a patient with the diagnosis of *functional pain*, or *psychogenic pain*, or, worst of all, *benign pain* does that patient great mental harm. The message to the patient is, "Your pain is not real," or "It's all in your head". Whenever a patient tells me that he or she has pain I have no doubt whatsoever that is true. Only the person

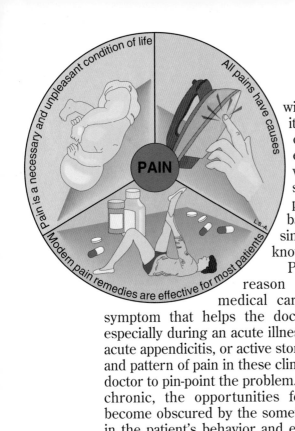

PAIN

Pain is a necessary and unpleasant condition of life

All pains have causes

Modern pain remedies are effective for most patients

L.S.A.

with the pain experiences it; not the doctor, or nurse, or spouse, or friend, or employer. We can see what the pain is doing to someone but it is not our pain, so we should not debase what the patient feels simply because we don't know what is causing it.

Pain is the most common reason for patients to seek medical care. It is an important symptom that helps the doctor make a diagnosis, especially during an acute illness such as heart attack, acute appendicitis, or active stomach ulcer. The location and pattern of pain in these clinical settings enables the doctor to pin-point the problem. When pain has become chronic, the opportunities for an exact diagnosis become obscured by the sometimes profound changes in the patient's behavior and emotions accompanying chronic pain. Patients are often misdiagnosed as having self-serving behavior and as seeking attention, sympathy, or financial reward. The reality is that the patient who has pain is very rarely faking (a malingerer) or obsessed with illness (a hypochondriac). In the vast majority of patients the experience of pain is a profound and often devastating personal crisis. Patients whose lives have been disrupted, whose marriages have failed, or who have lost their jobs because of pain, need compassion, understanding, and help to restore their well-being. Doctors who treat patients in pain owe it to them to believe exactly what is heard and not to place a value judgment on their painful experiences.

3. Modern pain remedies are effective for most patients.

For many patients there is no respite from pain. Studies from around the world – Australia, Europe, and North America, all sophisticated cultures with access to the most modern up-to-date drugs and techniques –

have repeatedly shown that seven of ten patients experience severe pain after surgery or from cancer. In other words, only thirty percent have adequate relief from pain, i.e., adequate from the patient's point of view. Doctors routinely underadminister pain-relieving medications even though they have been taught that they are effective when given in the full therapeutic dose. If only these potent analgesic drugs were used properly, patients could be free of severe, unrelenting pain. Failure by doctors to respond to a patient in obvious pain, distress, and suffering is a serious breach of medical ethics. The reason given most often for this failure is fear of legal liability should a complication arise through the prescription of high doses of strong analgesics. This makes no sense. No patient has sued his doctor for relieving his pain.

Outdated attitudes about strong analgesic drugs such as morphine, concerns over the potential risks of addiction and respiratory depression, concerns over abuse of controlled drugs, and a widespread lack of knowledge and understanding about pain by both doctors and nurses, have all contributed to the routine denial to patients of the relief they deserve. Upon graduation from medical school, doctors take the Hippocratic oath which has been their code of conduct for more than two thousand years. In this oath new doctors promise to alleviate suffering, to respect their patients, and to do no harm. It is obvious that at least the first of these promises is not always fulfilled. Through better understanding of what pain is and more aggressive use of effective treatments, the avoidable suffering and needless anguish of the victims of pain will become a thing of the past and we will then indeed have conquered pain.

The Prescription for Conquering Pain

A prescription is a set of instructions to your pharmacist to dispense treatment, usually in the form of a drug, and instructions to you on how to take it. There is no contract that says this prescription will relieve your problem even when you follow the instructions faithfully. The prescription is only a piece of paper with a message written on it. The message is very clear, if you can read your doctor's writing, but it is what you do with the message that is important.

The prescription for conquering pain is also a message to you if you suffer from pain. The message to you is:

*"If you know how, and want to,
you can conquer your pain."*

There is also a message to your doctor and to all future generations of doctors. This message is:

*"If you want to help your patients
who have pain, you'd better learn more
about how to do it well."*

There is also a message to your family, employer, and friends if you suffer from pain. This message is:

"It is not my fault that I have pain."

All of us can help conquer pain by changing our attitudes toward it, by learning more about it, by supporting more research into it, and by finding more effective ways to deal with it.

We usually think of conquering as a way of overpowering an enemy. Pain is the enemy within all of us, ever ready to break out and threaten our well-being. To conquer it is to know its weakness, and our strength.

Pain and Suffering

S uffering is distinct from pain. Suffering may be caused by pain that is severe, but for two people with similar pain, one may suffer while the other does not. Usually suffering arises when pain is perceived as something that will be never-ending or is due to some dire cause. Often suffering can be relieved when the cause of pain is known and can be corrected. However, suffering can also persist after pain has been completely relieved because of the anticipation that it will return. A good definition of suffering is *"distress due to the threat of loss of intactness of self from whatever cause"*.

The essence of suffering, like pain, is that it is entirely a personal experience – related to the *person* and not to his or her physical being. Although we can share the sense of suffering in a loved one, it is still an individual experience. It also profoundly tests the meaning of life. People who are suffering will say, "Why must this happen?" or, "This is no life for anyone".

The major distinction between pain and suffering is

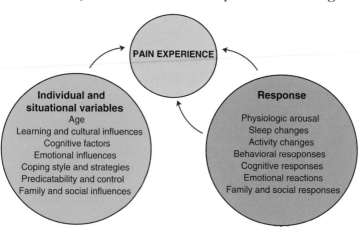

PAIN EXPERIENCE

Individual and situational variables
Age
Learning and cultural influences
Cognitive factors
Emotional influences
Coping style and strategies
Predicatability and control
Family and social influences

Response
Physiologic arousal
Sleep changes
Activity changes
Behavioral resoponses
Cognitive responses
Emotional reactions
Family and social responses

L.S.-A.

that pain is an unpleasant emotional and sensory experience that is closely linked to the past through previous exposure to pain; whereas suffering is a more conceptual emotion that is linked to the future through our fears of loss of self and purpose. There are similarities however, between suffering and pain, in that each causes disturbance of social, physical, and psychological well-being. Also, patients often hide their suffering or disguise their pain because to expose them makes them seem weak or vulnerable.

Until the 1980s few doctors specialized in pain management. Most doctors and nurses believed themselves perfectly capable of judging when a patient was having "real pain" and of deciding if pain medication was needed. Pain has not been considered a serious medical problem but simply a feature of a medical problem. Even today, treatment is generally aimed at the underlying cause of the problem rather than the pain itself. This approach sometimes works well if the cause of the problem is obvious, and the degree of pain that the patient has is close to what the doctor or nurse expects. For example, a sprained ankle is moderately painful, causes swelling, and makes walking difficult. Treatment usually includes strapping the ankle to provide support and limit further swelling. Anti-inflammatory drugs are prescribed to reduce the inflammation causing the pain. For most patients the problem is resolved within a week or two. Suffering is minimal in these circumstances. But there are some patients who continue to experience moderate to severe pain – pain that is not relieved by anti-inflammatory or other pain medications. This persistent pain takes on more threatening features and can cause great suffering. There is increased activity in the part of the body's nervous system related to the sympathetic nerves. These are the nerves that cause blood vessels to constrict,

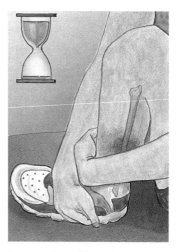
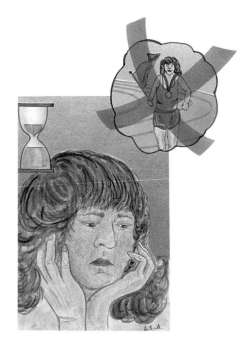

increasing blood pressure and restricting circulation. The heart beats faster and metabolism, hormone production, and kidney function are impaired. These "injury responses" are harmful and, if not treated properly, can lead to severe blood vessel spasms which, in rare cases, may even cause gangrene and require amputation of the limb. This is a dreadful outcome of such a simple injury as a sprained ankle. Proper attention to the treatment of the pain as well as the underlying causes of the pain will almost always ensure a speedy and full recovery.

The major difficulty with pain due to injury or disease is that the degree of pain is not always related to the degree of injury or seriousness of the disease. It seems logical that severe injuries should be very painful and minor injuries should not. Unfortunately it is not that simple. Experience with severe combat injuries or severe sports injuries has told us that these injuries are often painless during the first few hours. Doctors who have witnessed victims of such injuries first hand believe that distraction blocks out the pain. Some hours later the full consequences and implications of the injury begin to appear and the victim then feels severe pain which follows a course of slow resolution. In contrast to injuries that occur in a very stressful situation, a simple injury such as catching your finger in a door is immediately very painful. There are no serious consequences of such an injury and the pain usually subsides fairly quickly.

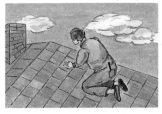

This distraction phenomenon is clearly evident in this true story of a man who was fixing some loose shingles on the roof of his one-storey house. Stretching to hold a shingle in place, he missed the nail and hit his hand with the hammer fracturing a bone. He described his pain as being severe immediately but becoming excruciating within a minute. Holding his injured hand against his body, he slithered across the roof to where he had placed the ladder. Unfortunately, before he could reach the ladder, he slipped off the roof and landed in a shrub below. He did not seriously injure himself in the fall but had some abrasions and cuts over his legs. He recalls clearly that from the moment he fell from the roof until some time later, he felt almost no pain in his injured hand. He does remember feeling very foolish when giving his history to the emergency room doctor an hour later.

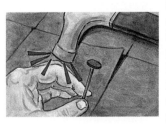

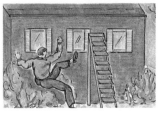

It is normal to focus on the external cause of pain rather than the pain itself, but if we wish to get long-lasting relief we have to accept that it is the pain that is most important. In other words, effective relief of pain begins with a full understanding of the pain. Early attention to the relief of pain

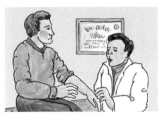

speeds recovery, reduces the risk of complications, and makes mobility easier. Most important, the reverse is also true. Inadequate pain relief delays recovery, increases the risk of complications, and prolongs inactivity. This turns what was a treatable acute problem into a chronic problem much more difficult to correct.

Pain is a universal experience. Both the smallest mouse and the largest elephant experience pain. Pain is not an "unmanly or unmacho" experience or a sign of weakness. It is purely subjective and is felt only by the person in pain. As witnesses we want to help. We imagine what the pain is like from what the victim tells us in words and gestures. Facial clues like a furrowed brow, a grimace, or crying; behavioral clues like inactivity or being withdrawn; postural clues like being bent over hugging the painful part, all become part of the impressions we build up of the patient in pain. Remember the child who holds up an injured finger so we can see the hurt. The child understands that the pain is in the hurt finger and has a clear image of this. We cannot see the hurt but we understand and console the child. Our impressions of someone in pain change with time and are affected by our biases and our own needs. For example, we may begin to question if the person is really in that much pain, or we may grieve that a loved one has such pain. This interaction between the person in pain and those who are witness to it often sets the direction of treatment and does not always benefit the victim.

The title of this book *Conquering Pain* implies that the elimination of pain is attainable, along with the elimination of suffering. The use of ineffective or unproven remedies for pain and inadequately trained care-givers are the main barriers to progress in conquering pain. These barriers must be removed. This may be an ambitious goal but advances in the methods of pain management during the past decade have been remarkable. In contrast, attitudes to pain have been much slower to change in response to this new knowledge of what pain is and how best to deal with it.

Patients need to know more about what their pain is. They know what it feels like, where it is, and what things make it worse or better. But there is nearly always an underlying concern or anxiety about why they are experiencing pain and what can be done to make it go away. This causes suffering. We need always to distinguish between pain and suffering. These two words are often used as if they convey the same idea, but

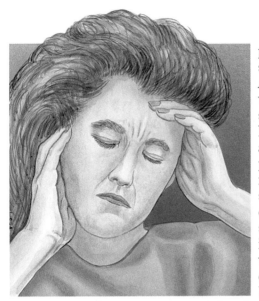

pain can occur without suffering and vice versa. Acute suffering can coincide with the onset of acute pain, such as the chest pains of a heart attack. But heart attacks are sometimes painless (silent) and there is no suffering. Chronic suffering without a great deal of pain occurs in several conditions, such as irritable bowel syndrome, where social and emotional disruption is distressful. Unrelieved pain nearly always causes mental and emotional suffering. Anxiety, depression, feelings of isolation, frustration, guilt, sadness, hopelessness, fear, anger, senses of loss or grief, despair, and abject loneliness are common in patients with chronic pain. The treatment of pain and of suffering requires different approaches often used together.

A patient asked recently "Have you any idea what it's like to have this much pain?" This man had been diagnosed with inoperable cancer of the bowel a couple of weeks before his referral to the clinic. Naturally he was angry. Naturally he was in severe pain. Naturally he wanted to get better; not just to have his pain taken away but to be made better by being relieved of his suffering. The possibility of a cure was out of the question but his was a cry for help much like a drowning man reaching up for a hand to pull him from certain oblivion. "No," I told him, "I do not know what it feels like to have your pain, but I understand fully the suffering your pain is causing you and I will do everything I can to remove it. I will also explain to you as best I can what your pain is, why you have it and what you can do to help it." Together we embarked on restoring a sense of intactness, comfort, and dignity to his life during his final months.

The Global Pain Epidemic

At the beginning of my medical career the pain problem was regarded as small-scale. I saw many patients every day who were sick or who needed surgery, but I don't recall that pain figured prominently for the doctors and nurses who attended them. There was compassion, but pain was something that was expected and when pain medication was prescribed everyone assumed that this would deal with it. In other words, there was no "pain problem" only some other problem, such as a broken bone, or inflamed bowel, or fibrositis, of which pain was but one part. Often there were so many patients to be attended to that less urgent cases waited their turn quietly, patiently, and most certainly in pain. We now know from surveys conducted by the World Health Organization that pain is the biggest single health problem anywhere. This global pain epidemic exceeds by far all other modern epidemics. Heart disease, lung disease, AIDS, muscular dystrophy, and parasitic diseases are worldwide health problems that afflict many millions of people; but daily pain, along with the resultant suffering, affects billions of people and is the leading cause of disability.

Modern Epidemics

Pain Epidemics

L.S.-A.

Recent epidemiological studies in the United States have provided reliable estimates of the size of the problem. Daily, twenty million Americans suffer moderate to severe pain from arthritis. Thirty million have persistent back pain and seven million of those are seriously disabled by pain. Millions more have muscle pains, headaches, chest pains, neck pains or pains in their arms or legs that

7

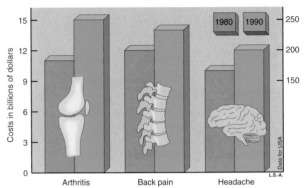

prevent them from doing such simple things as brushing their teeth or walking. If we relate these numbers to a world-wide scale there are probably 10 billion people who have pain from arthritis and as many as 15 billion who have back pain.

The cost of this pain epidemic is enormous. Total costs of drugs, other treatments, loss of work, and disability have been estimated to amount to between one-tenth and one-fifth of the global economy. In 1979 *The Washington Post* reported the estimated number and cost of lost workdays from lower back pain at 250 million workdays at a cost of 12 billion dollars. When all days lost through pain were totalled they reached nearly 2 billion workdays for a total cost of 75 billion dollars every year. Converted into 1994 dollars, the cost would have been well over 100 billion dollars. There is a need for more accurate data on the size and scope of the pain problem and how this translates into lost health. Evaluation of the costs of the treatment of pain has become a necessary fact of life for most health directorates in the industrialized world as a means of controlling expenses. But this does not tackle the problem of pain. It merely addresses the problem of containing the costs of dealing with it. We need to know much more about all aspects of pain and to promote effective programs that address preventative strategies and early injury recovery while ensuring better access to them. The most advanced and most widely available pain management programs are in North America and these have been shown to be cost-effective. However, in most parts of the world these services and programs are not available. The scarcity of pain management clinics staffed with well-trained physicians and therapists, even in some developed nations, means that access is restricted and usually involves a waiting period of many months or years before assessment and therapy can begin.

CHAPTER THREE

Knowing Your Pain

The reasons some people experience more pain than others give us insight into the nature of this beast. Children born with a rare abnormality – "congenital insensitivity to pain" – do not feel pain even when they injure themselves. Many lose fingers and toes from severe burns they do not feel. Yet their sense of touch is preserved. These children lack the type of nerves that carry painful messages from injured tissues to the brain. In leprosy, tissues, including nerves, are destroyed painlessly. All of the rest of us have these nerves and we experience pain 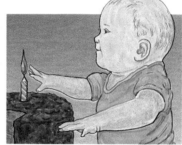 when we are injured but we each experience this sensation in different ways. We know of several factors that influence the way the pain system works:

Stress

To many doctors pain and stress are the by-products of unhealthy environments and lifestyles. The industrialized nations have altered the environment making it distinctly unhealthy through pollution of the air we breathe, the water we drink, and the soil in which we grow our food. The pace of modern life adds tremendous physical and mental stress. Coping with life has become a major health problem for many people. But when we look closely at statistics on the relation between lifestyle and environment and pain, these do not seem to be major factors. One survey shows that in a group of patients with chronic nondisabling pain, one in three exercises regularly, seven of ten do not smoke or drink alcohol to excess, and two of three eat a balanced, healthy diet. However, almost all of this group

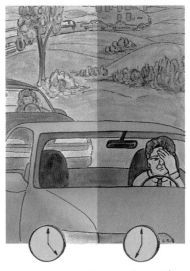

of patients report that stress is the most important factor aggravating their pain and preventing them from coping with it adequately. Few of these patients perceive stress as the *cause* of their pain.

Stress can be external and internal. External stress is forced on the individual by the environment: the demanding boss, being stuck in traffic and missing an important appointment, or the numerous other daily frustrations that can make some people feel as if they are constantly under duress. Internal stress is caused by feelings or sensations that one finds unpleasant or hurtful. Pain causes internal stress which can increase the intensity of the painful experience. External stress also aggravates pain. When people are asked to rate stress in their lives, those who report the most stress are also much more likely to have recurrent or chronic pains. Twice the number of people in the high stress group have menstrual pains, joint pains, back pains, and muscle pains, and three times the number have headaches and dental pain compared to a low stress group.

Incidence of Pain Related to Stress in Healthy People

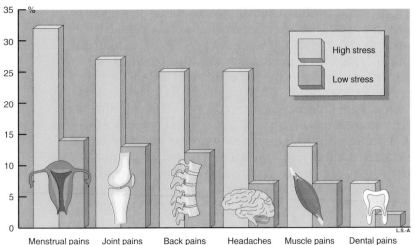

Does stress cause pain or is pain sensitized by stress? All the evidence points to stress as an aggravating factor but not as a cause of pain. To take this one step further, it is the body's response to stress that increases the perception or awareness of pain. A minor pain that in ordinary circumstances might hardly be noticed can become very hurtful if chronic stress is present. Stress causes the body to increase the production of catecholamines or "stress chemicals". These include adrenaline (epinephrine), noradrenaline (norepinephrine), serotonin, and dopamine. These chemicals are essential for the body's control of the cardiovascular system of the heart and blood vessels, of the kidneys which produce and excrete urine, of the intestine from which the body's nourishment comes, of hormones that balance the endocrine system, and of metabolism in the liver and other organs.

Stress increases the levels of these chemicals throughout the body. Centers in the brain respond to increased levels of catecholamines by sending out signals along the sympathetic nerves – to the heart, increasing the heart rate; to the blood vessels causing constriction and making the skin feel cold and sweaty and increasing blood pressure; and to other vital organs, altering their function. Muscles tense up, the heart races, and the tissues do not receive enough blood and begin to ache. Activation of these sympathetic nerve reflexes also connects to tissues that may have been injured, causing pain. The sympathetic nerves drive the injured tissue to sensitize the pain signals traveling up to the brain. This greatly increases the pain. When the sympathetic nerves are on overdrive during overwhelming acute stress, pain perception is blocked out temporarily because of distraction. Patients need to take charge of their stress to reduce the pain they feel. Often distraction techniques help them do this. In other words, when you are preoccupied with stress management you will feel less pain.

Under the Weather

Tension headaches, migraine, backaches, joint pains

and muscle pains are all aggravated by changes in the weather. In 1879, Dr. J.T. Everett of Sterling, Illinois, presented a paper to the Chicago Medical Association on his studies "in relation to the production of pain by the weather". For twelve years, beginning in 1866, Dr. Everett examined the records of the United States Signal Service, which monitored weather throughout Illinois, and documented the amount of pain felt by all the patients in his large practice. He was able to show a remarkable correlation between storm activity and increased pain, especially in those with chronic rheumatism. Any patient with arthritis, or tendinitis, or indeed any condition where inflammation of the tissues is present, will tell you that their pain increases just before a change in the weather. Why does a change in the weather cause pain to increase? Animals sense the coming storm and seek shelter before they need it. Is it anxiety or fear that provokes this protective behavior? One clue to the answer to this puzzle is that drugs that interfere with the functions of the sympathetic nerves can block this increase in pain when the weather changes. So it might be a subtle form of stressful signal, perhaps a change in atmospheric pressure, that stimulates the body's sympathetic responses enough to increase pain.

Aging

At birth we have already been provided with the apparatus needed to feel pain. Throughout our lives we make constant adaptations in the way we respond to damaging stimuli. It is ironic that as medical care has advanced and nutrition has improved, people are living longer but are suffering more pain. Osteoarthritis (inflamed joints) and painful osteoporosis (loss of calcium and softening of the bones) are diseases of aging. Symptoms of stiffness and pain in the joints usually appear around age 50 and progress slowly during the remainder of life. Most people can now expect to survive past age 75, so that the arthritis patient has to contend with at least a quarter of a century of daily pain.

The aging population is also more likely to develop cancer which is an increasingly more common cause of death in the elderly. If you live long enough, you are bound to die of something that a few decades ago would have been quite rare. Seven of ten cancer patients experience severe pain. However not all patients with advanced cancer experience pain. For the cancer patient, suffering has many dimensions, but fear of pain is the most important. Studies have shown that the degree of pain experienced after surgery, and the amount of analgesic drugs like morphine needed to relieve pain, steadily reduce as we get older. After major joint surgery, such as total hip-joint replacement, many elderly patients report very low levels of pain and require almost no analgesic medication. Yet these same patients would have had prolonged, and usually severe, hip pain prior to surgery. It seems that the pain that is felt acutely, such as after injury or surgery, lessens as we age; but the pain that has become chronic stays remarkably unchanged throughout life.

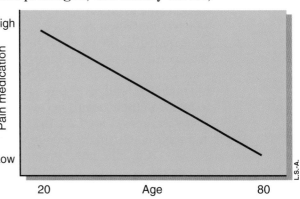

Poverty

The poor are more likely to develop chronic pain; but the explanation for this is complex as chronic pain also contributes to poverty. Patients are often made poor as a result of their pain. The three "Ds" of chronic pain are *distress*, *disability*, and *destitution*. The three "Rs" of treatment are *relief*, *recovery*, and *restoration*. Patients who have been injured at work, in traffic accidents, or through violence, often have severe pain that responds to appropriate treatment. But estimates show that one in five injured patients go on to have persistent pain. When the socio-economic status of the patient is factored in, the incidence of chronic pain in the well-to-do is no more than one in fifteen whereas the incidence in the poor is almost one in two.

Most types of heart, lung, intestinal, and endocrine disease have been linked to relative poverty. It is widely accepted that the richer you are the more likely you will be able to afford the best of health care, will be better nourished, will have better shelter, and will be much less likely to be exposed to the risk of disease. Actually, wealthy people are more likely to develop painful gout because of their lifestyles. Poverty imposes severe restrictions on health which are compounded by other significant variables including an inability or difficulty among those in need to take charge of their lives. There appear to be marked differences in the success of rehabilitation from injury in those who are steadily employed and those who do not work and who receive welfare continuously. The worker is more likely to be determined to recover and return to full employment – the worker has something to look forward to and something is missing when he or she is disabled. The unemployed tend, over time, to opt out and allow others to make all their health decisions for them. Under these circumstances, they lack the motivation to take charge and their pain usually becomes chronic.

It is the dilemma of social scientists who have examined the problem of poverty and the burden of pain that relieving poverty does not always solve the problem. It is difficult to change the attitudes and behavior of the patient who is poor and in pain. This dilemma definitely should not prejudice efforts to correct the situation, however.

Gender

Two-thirds of the patients referred to pain clinics are female. Does this mean that women have more pain?

Clinical studies have found that the level of pain experienced by women is significantly higher than that experienced by age-matched men for some types of pain but not for others. Fibromyalgia (fibrositis), a chronic painful muscle disorder, is as much as ten times more common in women than in men. Migraine, abdominal intestinal pain, pelvic pain, and back pains are up to three times more common in women compared to men. It seems that women do indeed have more pains.

Various theories have been proposed to explain this. One is that the pain apparatus (pain receptors in the tissues, nerve pathways, and brain centers) is fundamentally different in men and women. Another theory is that the differences in hormones between women (estrogen and progesterone) and men (testosterone) cause different sensitization of receptors so that women respond to low-level stimulation and men to high-level stimulation. Whatever the explanation (and at the present time it is unclear) it is almost certainly a biological not a psychological one.

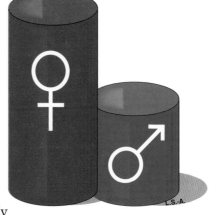

Elderly patients most commonly experience pain related to wear and tear on muscles and joints or the weakening pain following shingles. Nearly all of these patients are women. Men do not live as long and, therefore, pain in the elderly is becoming mainly a medical problem of women. At the other end of the age scale, chronic pelvic pain is almost exclusively a disorder in women. Premenstrual syndrome (PMS), primary dysmenorrhoea (painful periods), endometriosis (proliferative lesions in the uterus and related structures), and undiagnosed chronic pelvic pain probably afflict one in five women between 20 and 30 years of age. Obviously there are major differences between the pelvic organs of men and of women. Those in women have a primary reproductive function and it seems that young women in modern society are more

15

likely to develop pelvic dysfunction and pain.

Race and Culture

People of different racial, ethnic, or cultural backgrounds respond differently to pain and their experience of pain also differs. A recent survey of Americans of European, African, Hispanic, and Asian backgrounds found remarkable differences in pain levels reported after similar types of surgical operations. There was also a parallel difference in the amount of medication required to alleviate their pain. European-Americans experienced less pain than the other groups. The prevalence of pain in different parts of the world follows similar trends. The problem with this type of study is that it ignores many other factors known to influence the pain experience. It does not mean that patients are more likely to complain of pain because of their race or cultural background. It simply means that the pain experience is influenced by these and other factors.

It is important for the doctor or nurse who is treating a patient for pain to consider those factors relevant to the pain and to work on those that can be changed. Nothing can be done about the patient's status – being a woman or being a man; being 90 years old; or being a member of a particular race – but there is a great deal that can be done to help a patient come to terms with his or her pain, to understand it, and to find the best way to control it.

CHAPTER FOUR

Pain Words: Yours and Your Doctor's

Your doctor uses different words than you do to describe your pain. You use words that describe what it feels like, whereas your doctor uses words that describe what type of pain it is. Only you know what your pain feels like, yet experience shows it is quite difficult for patients to describe their pain clearly and in ways that others, let alone their doctor, might understand. The pain terms your doctor uses are unfamiliar and sometimes difficult to say but they are important because they help in diagnosing the cause of your pain.

What the Doctor Says and What It Means

Pain: an unpleasant sensory and emotional experience associated with actual or potential tissue damage, or described in terms of such damage.

Allodynia (al'oh'dinia): pain due to a stimulus which does not normally provoke pain.

Analgesia (an'al'geezia): absence of pain in response to stimulation which would normally be painful.

Analgesic: a substance or drug relieving pain.

Anodyne: anything that relieves pain or soothes.

Anesthesia Dolorosa (an'ess'theezia/doll'or'rosa): pain in an area which is anesthetic (numb).

Central Pain: pain associated with a lesion in the central nervous system (brain or spinal nerves).

Dysesthesia (diss'ess'theezia): an unpleasant abnormal sensation whether spontaneous or evoked.

Hyperesthesia (hi'per'ess'theezia): increased sensitivity to stimulation, excluding the special senses of vision, hearing, and taste.

Hyperalgesia (hi'per'al'geezia): an increased

17

response to a stimulus which is normally painful.

Hyperpathia (hi'per'path'ia): an increased response to a stimulus, and increased threshold.

Hypoalgesia (hi'po'al'geezia): diminished pain in response to a normally painful stimulus.

Hypoesthesia (hi'po'ess'theezia): a decreased sensitivity to stimulation, excluding the special senses of vision, hearing, and taste.

Neuralgia (new'raal'gia): pain in the area of the body served by a nerve or nerves.

Neuritis (new'rye'tiss): inflammation of a nerve or nerves.

Neuropathy (new'raw'pathy): a disturbance of function or pathological change in a nerve.

Nociceptor (no'see'septor): a receptor specifically sensitive to a tissue-damaging stimulus.

Noxious (nox'yus): a stimulus that is damaging to normal tissues.

Pain Threshold: the least experience of pain which a subject can recognize.

Pain Tolerance Level: the greatest level of pain which a subject is prepared to tolerate.

Paresthesia (parr'ess'theezia): an abnormal sensation, whether spontaneous or caused by an external stimulation.

What the Patient Says

The words you might use to describe your pain have been assembled in several types of pain questionnaires. The most widely used was developed by a Montreal psychologist, Dr. Ronald Melzack. It is the McGill Pain Questionnaire and contains three classes of words – sensory, affective, and evaluative – that patients use to describe their experience of pain.

Sensory words describe the feelings or sensations of pain and are divided into ten subcategories:
•**Temporal words**: flicking, quivering, pulsing, throbbing, beating, pounding
•**Spatial words**: jumping, flashing, shooting
•**Punctate pressure words**: pricking, boring, drilling,

stabbing, lancing
- **Incisive pressure words**: sharp, cutting, lacerating, spreading, radiating, penetrating, piercing
- **Constrictive pressure words**: pinching, pressing, gnawing, tight, numb, drawing, squeezing, tearing, cramping, crushing
- **Traction pressure words**: tugging, pulling, wrenching
- **Thermal words**: hot, burning, scalding, searing, cool, cold, freezing
- **Brightness words**: tingling, itchy, smarting, stinging
- **Dullness words**: dull, sore, hurting, aching, heavy
- **Miscellaneous words**: tender, taut, rasping, splitting

Affective words describe the emotional experience of pain in five categories:
- **Tension words**: tiring, exhausting
- **Autonomic words**: sickening, suffocating
- **Fear words**: fearful, frightful, terrifying
- **Punishment words**: punishing, gruelling, cruel, vicious, killing
- **Miscellaneous words**: wretched, blinding

Evaluative words describe the severity of pain and include:
- **Anchor words**: mild, discomforting, distressing, horrible, excruciating
- **Synonyms**: annoying (nagging), troublesome (nauseating), miserable (agonizing), intense (dreadful), unbearable (torturing)

These 83 words cover the vocabulary that patients use to describe what their pain feels like. The doctor knows what these words mean and the feelings they convey. Careful use of these terms *should* produce a better understanding of your problem. Unfortunately, few doctors take the time to document in detail the word description a patient gives of his or her pain. There is a tendency for doctors to want only to know where the pain is and how bad it is. These are also the priorities of many patients. It is as if the only thing the patient wants is for the doctor to get on with it and do something about it quickly. However, for complicated pains or for chronic pains, these descriptor words are important in making a diagnosis and providing appropriate treatment.

Although some patients are quite comfortable describing their pain to the doctor, most patients, at least on the initial visit, will understate their pain. Often there is a sense of seeking approval from the doctor when the treatment prescribed has not worked in the way hoped for or expected. Even when asked by a friend or co-worker, "How are you today?" most of us will simply reply "Oh, fine". Even though we may be in considerable pain, we don't want to be a bother.

Specialists in pain management find that patients give much more useful information when questions are put directly. When you speak about your pain you should use the best word descriptors you can to describe what your pain feels like and what it is doing to you. The doctor may say, "Tell me about your pain from the beginning". If your response is, "My family doctor thinks I have a slipped disc," you are deflecting the doctor's question to what you think is the cause of your pain rather than the pain itself. I have never seen a slipped disc nor do I believe such a thing exists, yet it is a phrase that is commonly used by patients who have back pain. I would then repeat, "Tell me about your pain". If the spouse is also present she might reply, "It happened when he fell at work, that's what the problem is". Again this avoids the question. Both the patient and the spouse think of his back pain in terms of injury rather than of the subjective pain experienced. It is almost always better for the doctor to listen to the story of how the injury happened and then come back to the original question. The patient will then describe what the pain felt like and where it was and relate any changes in the character of the pain between its onset and the time of examination.

The more your doctor knows about your pain the better. But a doctor only hears what you have to tell so be as specific as you can. Don't expect your doctor to have *all* the answers to your problem. However, you should expect that your doctor knows something about pain and how to treat it effectively. The best doctor will guide you to an awareness and acceptance of taking responsibility for your own health, including your pain. If you have chronic pain you should concentrate on overcoming what your pain is doing to you and certainly not let it run your life. Being able to *communicate* your feelings is a very important part of gaining control.

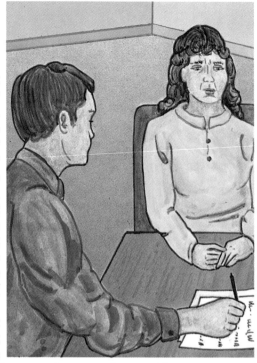

Some patients cannot use words or find great difficulty speaking, such as those who have had a stroke or who were born with cerebral palsy. For them the doctor uses other ways to interpret what they wish to communicate. The doctor may say, " I am going to ask you a series of questions about your pain and if you agree squeeze my finger". The questions are very direct: "Is your pain here?", "Does it move to there?", "Does it keep you awake?", etc. Having the patient hold the doctor's finger is a simple and effective means of literally connecting to the patient who cannot speak or who has difficulty speaking.

A patient who has cerebral palsy arrived for a routine follow-up clinic visit with a notice taped to her wheelchair. The notice was neatly printed in her own hand and must have involved great effort to write out. It said: "I am not retarded or stupid. I have a neurological condition called cerebral palsy that makes it difficult for me to speak. Thank you". This patient was obviously only too aware that others, seeing her struggle to express herself, misread completely what was wrong with her. Sometimes this same kind of misinterpretation occurs when patients who are experiencing a great deal of pain and suffering are unable to convey to those around them exactly what they are going through.

When the lack of a common language prevents communication a competent interpreter should accurately translate exactly what is said by the patient and the doctor. Children are usually thought to be unable to communicate their painful experiences except, in a very primitive way, by crying. This is wrong. Most children who are past the toddler stage can express themselves clearly when they have pain. If the doctor or nurse is prepared to listen the child will usually comply.

Measuring Pain

There are several simple and reliable methods for assessing the severity of pain. These use either words or signs to enable the patient to judge how bad the pain is so that the doctor has a more exact record of the pain.

These verbal scales use numerical scores to describe pain. 0 = no pain, 1 = a little pain, 2 = some pain, 3 = a lot of pain, 4 = the worst pain possible. In another variation the patient assigns a number to pain.

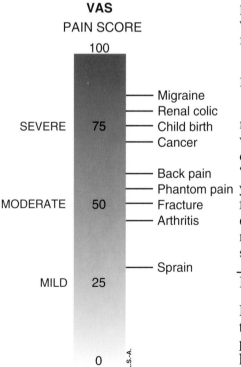

VAS

PAIN SCORE

	100
SEVERE	75
MODERATE	50
MILD	25
	0

— Migraine
— Renal colic
— Child birth
— Cancer

— Back pain
— Phantom pain
— Fracture
— Arthritis

— Sprain

L.S.-A.

0	5	10
No pain	Some Pain	Worst Pain

The most widely used measurement method uses no words but only a line 10 centimeter long called the "visual analog scale" on which you mark a point where you feel your pain lies. The distance from zero is measured and converted into a score in millimeters.

No pain	Worst pain

For example, if your pain on the VAS is 80 you have severe pain but if the VAS is 15 you have mild pain.

Your Mind and Your Pain

P ain is a complex and distressing psychological experience. Most patients, however, tend to want to focus on their physical symptoms. After all, the pain is usually felt in a part of the body they can see. For example, when you have a headache and look in the mirror, what you see is your head and it is easy to visualize that something must be wrong inside. This process of describing pain in a physical way is called *somatization*. Psychiatrists use this term when they feel that a patient is expressing what are essentially psychological effects in terms of the physical part of the body (the soma) where they feel their pain to be, or as other bodily symptoms. When pain is severe and prolonged, the mental anguish and emotional distress that accompany it can produce even more suffering than the pain itself.

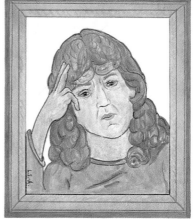

There are two types of psychological reaction to pain – emotional and behavioral. These reactions are important in acute pain situations but in chronic pain they may be the *only* important features. There is considerable misunderstanding about these psychological aspects of pain by many patients and their doctors. It is as if these emotional effects and changes in behavior somehow intrude upon and distort the picture portrayed by the patient who is having pain and the one perceived by the doctor. This makes diagnosis very difficult and often leads to inappropriate management through under-treatment or over-treatment with mood-

23

altering drugs. Your doctor must be fully aware of the key role of these psychological reactions to pain and provide early and effective treatment; otherwise, your treatable acute pain could progress to a chronic type that may be very difficult to treat.

Emotional Responses

Pain is never emotionally neutral. All patients, whatever their age or circumstances, experience some distress when they are in pain. Arousal of emotions and distress has a focal point of fear and feelings of helplessness – fear that your pain means something is very seriously wrong in your body. Perhaps you think it might be cancer, or that it might cause paralysis and

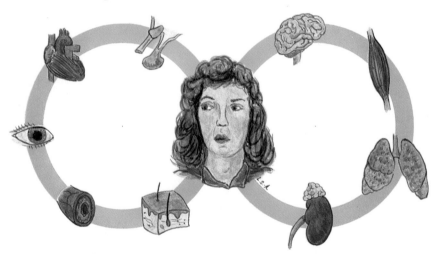

permanent disability. Fear can become dread that your pain might progressively worsen. This can make you literally sick with fear. Helplessness comes from the feeling that your body is no longer yours and that your pain has taken control of all your feelings and activities preventing you from being yourself. It might seem that no matter how hard you try, the pain is there ahead of you pushing you back. Your normal healthy sense of well-being retreats into a distant past, leaving you with little to look forward to and very little to comfort you.

These emotional reactions can, and usually do,

increase the sensitivity of injured tissues making your pain worse. Your pain then feeds on your anxiety which in turn feeds on your pain. The more distressed you become the more you will become depressed, which further adds to your mental anguish. We know that some emotional reactions are triggered by the release of chemicals in the brain and that anxiolytic (anxiety-relieving) and anti-depressant drugs reduce distress and pain at the same time.

When a patient has acute pain, two things must be considered after the likely cause of pain has been determined: first, how can the pain be relieved? and second, how can health and well-being be restored? Most often this means that both pain-relieving and anxiety-relieving medication will be administered. If the patient has chronic pain the emotional responses are likely to be much more complex. Depression, morbid thoughts, even suicidal thoughts, lead to a semivegetative state in some patients. Activity decreases to minimal levels and patients simply lose interest in themselves and their surroundings. Weight gain is usual which further adds to depression and inactivity. Such patients truly have a disease called chronic pain.

Behavioral Responses

The behavioral responses to pain are the movements, postures, and body expressions we use when we are experiencing pain. These are the features your doctor observes and uses to assess whether your pain is severe, appropriate to what is wrong with you, and as a gauge to planned therapy. We have all seen someone in pain, showing facial expressions or other aspects of "pain body-language", such as a hunched up posture, standing or sitting stiffly, or bracing or rubbing the painful area. You will almost always do the same thing if you have pain. These behaviors are a way of letting others know how much pain you are having without the bother, and for many patients the embarrassment, of telling them. Many studies have demonstrated that doctors and nurses are more likely to respond to such behaviors and administer pain-relieving medication. However, relying on these behavioral expressions alone to decide on therapy results in many patients not receiving adequate relief. Ironically those who moan and groan the loudest will likely receive prompt attention and be given relief.

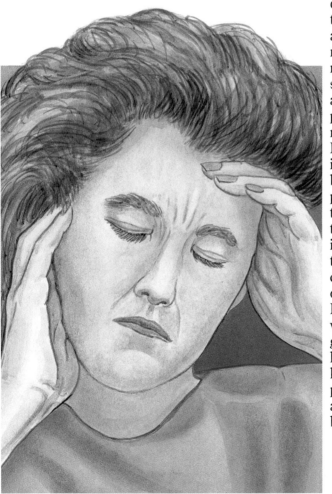

CHAPTER SIX

The Pain Map

Understanding pain depends upon knowing how pain signals are generated, how they travel from one part of the body to another, and what connections are made along the way. Just as a good road map is helpful when we want to travel through an unfamiliar part of the country, a *pain map* shows what pathways pain signals take, what centers are visited, and where the final destination lies. The pain map represents the three components of the pain system in the body – *sensors*, *circuits*, and *switches*.

Pain Sensors

Painful stimuli are detected by tissue sensors called *nociceptors*. These sensors are found throughout the body in skin, muscles, ligaments, bones, internal organs, and even the brain. They represent the early warning system signalling that something has caused, or is about to cause, damage to the tiny cells of body tissues. The sensors are stimulated into action mainly by heat, mechanical stress, or irritant chemicals. At each ending of the sensory nerves which are only one-one hundred thousandth of a centimeter in diameter, there are an estimated 10,000 to 100,000 nociceptors for each nerve fiber. This means that there are billions of nociceptors for every square centimeter of body tissue. Your body is completely saturated with pain sensors that are normally fairly quiet, but ready to deliver signals to your central nervous system when aroused.

There are at least six different types of pain sensor

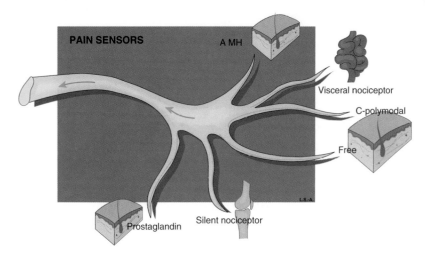

PAIN SENSORS
A MH
Visceral nociceptor
C-polymodal
Free
L.S.-A.
Prostaglandin Silent nociceptor

and the density and mix of these varies among different tissues. This means that activation of nociceptors by surgery on the uterus, for example, produces a quite different set of pain signals to the signals generated after bone surgery. The chemical stimulation of pain sensors is particularly important with tissue damage from inflammation, surgery, or extreme changes in metabolism. These chemicals include *prostaglandins* produced at the site of tissue damage, *histamine* released from granular cells (mast cells) involved in inflammatory reactions, *bradykinin* from blood proteins released when small blood vessels are damaged, and *serotonin* from blood cells (platelets) which are important for blood clotting. When the pain sensors are activated by any of these chemicals they are triggered in sequence (nociceptor recruitment). The intensity of signals increases as more and more sensors are stimulated. This causes intense irritation of small nerve endings and rapid firing in the pain circuits.

Pain Circuits

The pain circuits are the pathways along which pain signals travel and the connections made enroute to the central nervous system (brain and spinal cord). Two types of nerve fiber conduct pain signals, in the form of electrical impulses (action potentials), to the brain. The first type is the A-delta fiber which has an insulated covering (myelin sheath) allowing the pain signals to travel very fast (5 to 15 meters per second) from one end of a fiber to another. These A-delta fibers carry signals that are felt as sharp pain that is easily localized, for example, when you touch a hotplate with the tip of your finger, pain signals travel rapidly to your brain registering that you have pain in your finger, and flashing to your hand to remove it from the heat. This all happens in a fraction of a second. The second type of fiber is the C-polymodal which has no myelin covering and is therefore uninsulated. Pain signals travel more slowly along the C-polymodal fibers at usually less than one meter per second. These fibers carry pain signals that are felt as dull or diffuse pain that is difficult to localize accurately, for example, most types of backache.

In acute pain both types of fiber are active, but in chronic pain it is mainly the C-polymodal fibers that carry pain signals. Both types of fiber carry signals toward the spine where the major nerve in the body, the spinal cord, is located and is protected by the bones that make up the spine. Carrying pain signals to the spinal cord these are called *afferent nerves.* Inside the spinal cord the afferent nerves, which consist of bundles of many millions of individual nerve fibers make connections with "second order nerves" in an area called the *substantia gelatinosa of the dorsal horn.* This is an area at the back of the spinal cord which has the consistency of 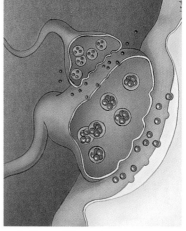 jelly. The connections between each of the afferent nerves and the second order nerves are such that the pain signals have to jump across a tiny space between the nerves called the *synaptic cleft.* They do this through the very rapid release of chemical transmitters that carry the electrical signal to the receiving surface membrane of the next nerve and so on, in sequence, to the brain. The most important of these transmitters are *substance-P, n-methyl-d-aspartate* and *glutamate.* Without the release of these chemicals, the signal would stop at the spinal ending of the primary afferent nerve and no pain would be felt. Multiple connections are made at upper levels in the spinal cord and at several levels in the brain within the afferent tracts (*ascending stimulatory pathway*). There are drugs available that have very specific actions at these connections in the spinal cord and the brain which modulate or block the transmission of pain signals to the central nervous system, thus diminishing or relieving pain.

Switches
Whenever pain signals are generated in the tissues and enter the central nervous system, the body switches on its *pain resistors.* There are several ways the body tries to prevent pain signals from activating all the pain circuits simultaneously. A pain resistor works like a dimmer switch that can gradually lower the level of light by inhibiting or resisting the electrical current flowing to a lamp.

Filtering the Signals
A filter separates pain signals as to their size (large or small), or significance (important or unimportant) and, depending on the characteristics of the filter, selects the signals that will be allowed to enter the pain circuits. In the tissues the various types of pain sensors (nociceptors) have different thresholds for firing. Having a threshold means that the intensity of stimulation has to reach a certain level before the full blown pain signal is generated. Small stimuli, below the threshold level, do not generate pain signals and none of the pain circuits are activated. It is possible for the firing threshold for nociceptors to move up or down depending on the circumstances. When the threshold is lowered (e.g., during increased tissue sensitivity associated with injury), pain signals are more easily generated not only by a less intense painful stimulation

but, most importantly, by stimuli that are not normally painful, such as touch. Conversely when the threshold is raised it takes much more intense stimulation before pain signals are produced. This happens in some patients with neuritis caused by diabetes or chronic alcoholism.

Because the different types of nociceptor respond only to particular forms of stimulation, some signals are allowed to dominate the receptor field crowding out other less intense or less important signals. This process is like having many interchangeable sieves to control the size of signals that can enter the next level in the pain circuit; the one with the largest pores allows all signals through, while the one with the smallest pores blocks most of the signals. By changing "sieves" to filter pain signals the body can, at any given time, open up or close down the movement of pain signals from their source to various levels in the central nervous system. What this means to you, if you are experiencing pain, is that the quality and intensity of that part of your pain relating to tenderness (acutely sensitive to touch) can suddenly change without warning.

Gating the Signals

In the central nervous system, gates in the pain circuits can be closed to block the passage of some signals, in much the same way you would close a garden gate to stop your dog running loose in the street. *The Gate Control Theory of Pain* described by Dr. Ronald Melzack, a psychologist, and Dr. Patrick Wall, a neurophysiologist, is a very useful starting point in understanding how pain signals can be modified to lessen the pain experienced. Remember that pain signals travel to the spinal cord by A-delta fibers (the fast route) and C-polymodal fibers (the slow route). Generally, signals that travel fastest have priority at the first "gate" in the dorsal horn of the spinal cord. The gate is wide open to pain signals traveling in A-delta fibers, but the gate is slammed shut to the more slowly moving signals traveling along the C-polymodal fibers. When the

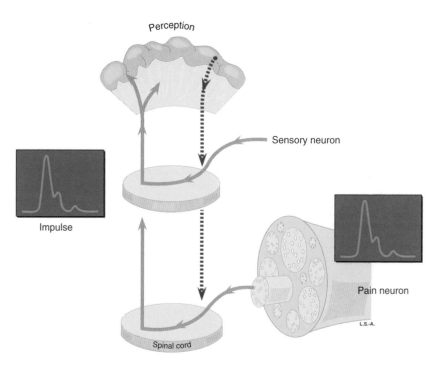

Perception

Sensory neuron

Impulse

Pain neuron

L.S.-A.

Spinal cord

A-delta pain signals reach the midbrain, a switch is activated that starts to close the gate to the A-delta pain signals and gradually opens up the gate to C-polymodal pain signals. Thus, when sharp intensely painful signals reach the midbrain, the gating of signals in the spinal cord changes the character (sharp to dull), location (localized to diffuse), and intensity (severe to less severe) of the pain experienced.

If you suffer from one of the many types of chronic pain, the gating of pain signals in your spinal cord probably only involves C-polymodal pain signals, since the sharp pain associated with the original injury or inflammation will usually have settled. There is a large (4 to 8 micrometers in diameter) very fast type of fiber (A-beta) in the skin that is not active in chronic pain but which connects to second order nerves in the dorsal horn. The A-beta nerves can be stimulated by small electrodes placed on the skin over the painful area. This stimulation causes the spinal gate to close to the passage of C-polymodal pain signals and some types of A-delta signals resulting in relief of pain. This technique is called *transcutaneous electrical nerve stimulation* (TENS). TENS produces relief of pain in some acute situations and in chronic pain by using secondary switches to block the entry of pain signals into the upper parts of the brain.

Secondary Switches

There are two important secondary means by which the central nervous system modifies and inhibits electrical activity in the pain circuits. The first is a descending set of nerves that arise in the part of the midbrain called the *thalamus* through which all pain signals reaching the midbrain must pass. Below the thalamus pain signals travel through the *reticular formation* where autonomic reflexes, like sweating and pallor (skin feels cold and looks pale), are provoked. There is a secondary gate in the thalamus that processes pain signals in two directions. The first goes directly to the uppermost or conscious part of the brain, the *cortex*, causing the "ouch" or withdrawal response. The second route travels through the *limbic system* and it is here that the emotional responses to severe pain arise. Above the thalamus pain signals enter an area of *sensory specific projections* on the cortex that tells you "your left index finger hurts" if that is the injured finger.

When pain signals travel to the thalamus they go through a channel called the periaqueductal grey matter lying immediately below it. Nerves in the *periaqueductal grey matter* descend to all levels of the spinal cord where they make con-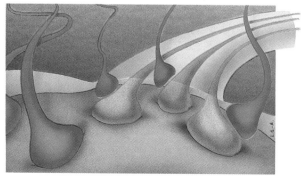nections with se-cond order nerves in the substantia gelatinosa of the dorsal horn. When these *descending inhibitory pathways* are activated by the arrival of pain signals in the midbrain, they inhibit the passage of pain signals in the dorsal horn. They do this by producing various chemicals next to the nerve cells that receive the pain signal. These chemicals (*noradrenaline, serotonin, gamma amino butyric acid [GABA], somatostatin,* and *glycine*) are produced along with a group of endogenous opioids (the body's own morphine-like substances), including *endorphins, enkephalins,* and *dynorphins.* When these inhibitory neurons are activated entry of painful impulses into the central nervous system is switched off. Less pain is experienced. When your doctor prescribes morphine or one of the other opiate drugs because you have severe pain, the relief you get depends on activation of the descending inhibitory pathways. New drugs have been developed to mimic this inhibition or block the release of specific transmitters for pain signals. The body can also increase the production of endorphins and activate the descending inhibitory pathways through exercise. For this reason, *exercise is an essential part of any pain management program.*

There is a very delicate but complex balance within the pain system between the forces driving pain signals in and the internal forces trying to expel or block these signals from disrupting your sense of "ease". No two patients are alike in the way this balance is struck or in how easily it may be tipped one way or the other. The important thing to recognize is that the body normally has a very effective system in place to protect your sense of ease. When this is disturbed, recovery is a matter of restoring this balance.

Sensitization

So far, we have seen the pain map as it relates to sensory nerves. But there is a second parallel group of nerves called *sympathetic afferents* that are part of the body's autonomic nervous system. The sympathetic and parasympathetic nerves conduct signals to and from all the body's organs, controlling their function. Sweat glands in the skin produce sweat in response to sympathetic nerve stimulation. When the sympathetic nerves are stimulated in the heart and major blood vessels, your heart rate and blood pressure increase. The movement of the intestine necessary for digestion is slowed by sympathetic stimulation.

The sympathetic afferent nerves also carry pain signals to the spinal cord. In fact, about half of all C-polymodal fibers that carry pain signals are sympathetic. Pain sensors (nociceptors) are also located at various sites along these sympathetic nerves. They are activated by similar changes in their environment as are the nociceptors on sensory nerve endings. The major difference between the activation of sympathetic nerves compared to sensory nerves is that activity in sympathetic nociceptors causes sensitization of neighboring nerves, including sensory branches. This causes a marked lowering of the threshold for activating pain impulses in afferent nerves of all types. For the patient this feels like an area of greatly increased sensitivity, where light stroking or even a draught of air can cause intense burning pain. Pain after shingles (herpes zoster) has this characteristic of increased sensitivity to light touch.

In the dorsal horn of the spinal cord a similar type of sensitization occurs which is called *spinal plasticity*. Hyperactive reflexes occur in the outgoing *efferent sympathetic nerves* connecting to the various organs of the body, as well as in *efferent motor nerves* to muscles, causing muscle spasms. These muscle spasms are in themselves painful. This further increases the pain experienced. In the tissues the outgoing (efferent) nerves and the ingoing (afferent) nerves are closely connected. Pain signals originating in one area of the body travel to the spinal cord causing pain and stimulating activity in efferent nerves going back to the area of pain. This closes the loop between input and output causing the pain to continue unabated even if the cause of the original painful signal is no longer present. To add to this circle of activity in the pain circuits, efferent impulses in sympathetic nerves can travel to areas of the body some distance away from where the original pain arose, causing localized, then spreading, burning pain. This type of pain is called *referred pain* because it is referred to another part of the body away from where the underlying problem exists.

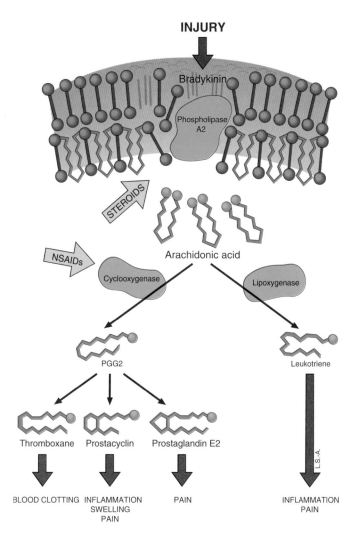

Sensitization in the tissues also increases when the prostaglandin group of compounds is produced following tissue injury or inflammation. These natural compounds are the most important mediators of the chemical basis of pain and are also important in inflammation. They are produced from *arachidonic acid* which is found on the surface of all living cells in the body. Release of arachidonic acid after injury requires the activation of bradykinin and an enzyme called *phospholipase A2*. Injections of cortisone or other steroid drugs block phospholipase A2 and prevent the release of arachidonic acid, and so reduce inflammation and pain. The metabolism of arachidonic acid requires two other enzymes – *cyclo-oxygenase*, and *lipoxygenase* which break down the arachidonic acid into several active compounds including prostaglandins (involved in inflammation and pain), prostacyclins (mainly involved in inflammation and changes in the blood vessels), thromboxanes (needed for normal blood clotting), and leukotrienes (also involved in pain and inflammation). These compounds, along with histamine, serotonin, and bradykinin, increase the sensitivity of pain sensors. Drugs like aspirin and other nonsteroidal anti-inflammatory drugs block the activity of cyclo-oxygenase cutting off the production of painful irritants like the prostaglandins. For this reason this class of drug is widely used for the treatment of painful chronic inflammatory conditions like arthritis.

Summary of the Pain Map

During acute pain, the pain map is volatile. Areas within the receptor field are rapidly subjected to forces that change the pattern, quality, and intensity of receptor activity. Pain circuits are also rapidly activated or shut down as the process of modulation of pain signals reaches a maximum. Once the receptor field is stabilized the signals and the circuits through which they travel become temporarily fixed through *templating*. This means that when the receptor field stops wobbling around, the central nervous system accepts this new equilibrium and tries to maintain it. Pain signals and the pattern of signal movement become directed along the best routes. When a new burst of activity arrives in the pain circuits, the inhibitory pathways, now already finely tuned, minimize any disturbance of the balance.

When pain does not go away within the expected time needed to resolve its underlying cause, pain has become chronic. Sometimes the change from acute to chronic pain occurs over a few weeks; but more often it takes several months. The conventional definition of chronic pain is one that has persisted for at least six months, but I prefer relating the term "chronic pain" to the expected recovery period from the acute episode. When pain becomes chronic the pattern of pain signals is firmly imprinted in the receptor field. The hills and valleys of the pain map are now very similar to a topographical map where elevation (height of the pain signals at that site) and distance (space between important features) can be visualized easily. In chronic pain the features on the pain map may change progressively but only very slowly. Sometimes a short burst of activity occurs when there is aggravation of pain but this usually will be quickly masked by the predominant pattern of the chronic features.

I am often asked why one patient may make an uneventful recovery after an injury, while another may not recover and may go on to develop chronic pain. There is no easy answer to this question. The circumstances of the injury may be virtually identical, yet the outcome may be vastly different. The answer likely has to do with the way individuals process the pain signals generated when an injury occurs. The important role of the *"higher centers"* of the brain, the capacity to switch on inhibitory pathways, and the ability to produce pain relieving endorphins, are undoubtedly crucial for those intent on preventing their acute pain from becoming chronic.

CHAPTER SEVEN

Taking Charge
of Your Pain

Y our start on the road to recovery begins when you take charge of your life with pain. Chronic pain makes it very difficult to know where to begin, but you must be determined not to let pain run your life. For many patients chronic pain is a disease far worse than any of the usual diseases.

I call chronic pain a disease because, like other diseases, something has taken away the normal feeling of comfort or ease. We can more fully understand the things we visualize. A black eye, a cut finger, or the swelling of a tumor gives us an idea what this "dis-ease" is. But when the dis-ease is no more than an "unpleasant sensory and emotional experience" which we call pain, how do we come to terms with its shadowy and harmful effects? The word *pain* comes from the Greek word *poine* meaning penalty or punishment. Many patients with pain do feel punished, and unjustly so. The opposite of pain is pleasure, which has been considered throughout history as the absence of any feelings of discomfort. People spend most of their lives seeking pleasure. This is the natural order of things which, if realized, brings happiness and contentment. When pain appears it disturbs this natural order and pleasure becomes an illusion. Without pain our life can be as full or as empty as we wish, dictated only by our own needs. When pain intervenes, we feel we no longer have control over our lives and experience a steady disintegration of self.

I could describe the history of any one of many thousands of patients to illustrate this disease of chronic pain, but one will suffice. I will call her "B" but I have changed very little of her story. She is thirty-two years old. She married her childhood sweetheart, "J", when she was eighteen. They had their first child, a daughter, two years later and a son one year after that. J had a good job as a manager of a printing firm, and when their son was two years old B began a well paid job in sales at a local department store. At this period in their lives both B and her husband were very active socially and in sports. Their daughter, aged ten, died suddenly from complications of meningitis. Over the next few months, with the help of a counselor, B successfully overcame her tragic loss and regained her health. Two years ago, she twisted her lower back while playing ball with her son. It had not hurt badly at the time but by evening she was having painful muscle spasms. She hardly slept that night and J took her to their family doctor the next day. The doctor examined her briefly and reassured her that nothing was very seriously wrong. He told her to go home and rest and gave her a prescription for a pain medication with codeine. He did warn her that the codeine might make her drowsy. She had instructions to call her doctor again in a week or two if her pain had not settled.

B did exactly as her doctor had advised and went to bed. The medication made her very drowsy but she persevered. After two weeks the pain was no better and seemed to have spread further up her back. She also felt increasingly weak and was having headaches which she very rarely had, apart for a time after her daughter died. She felt more and more unwell and was sure that there must be something making her feel so miserable. Her doctor examined her and found that her muscles were indeed weak and she had lost much of her muscle bulk. Previously she had been very fit and had excellent muscle tone. Now her muscles were quite lax. Arrangements were made for some tests including x-rays of her back, an EMG (electromyograph) to test her muscles, and blood tests. These required three weeks to arrange and get results. In the meantime she continued to go downhill and gradually lost the energy to do even the lightest chores around the house. The department store wrote to say that they could not hold her job open for more than a further two weeks. When she visited her doctor she was told that nothing showed up in the tests and he was still convinced there was nothing to worry about. Clearly, from her view, there was a great deal to worry about. She was rapidly becoming an

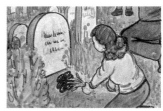

invalid and her relationship with her husband, once very close, was becoming distant. In short, all the pleasure in her life had disappeared. To satisfy B's insistence that there must surely be something someone could do to find out what was wrong and sort it out, her doctor arranged for her to see an orthopedic surgeon (a specialist in bone and joint surgery) who told her she had a

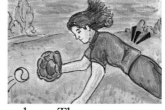

mechanical back but didn't explain what this was. She next saw a rheumatologist (a specialist in bone and joint diseases) who wondered whether she might be developing fibrositis, which was explained as a kind of inflammation in the ligaments of her back. He could not offer treatment except to advise her to try to relax as she seemed quite tense. She was seen next by a gynecologist because her

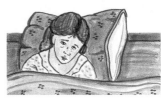

menstrual periods had become irregular. The gynecologist could find nothing wrong but said she would like to see B in six months if she was not improving.

From the time she twisted her back to her visit with the gynecologist more than a year had passed. B had long ago lost her job. She was physically infirm. Most movements were painful. Her pain was

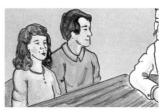

now all over her back. She had severe headaches every day. Sometimes the pain would shoot into her legs. Their social life together was nonexistent but J, who felt he had to get away from the oppressive atmosphere around the house, saw his friends regularly. B became depressed and even had thoughts of taking her own life. Her doctor arranged an urgent consultation with a psychiatrist.

At first B felt this was the final rejection of her back problem as something that she was just imagining. Her psychiatrist found that B had considerable anxiety, clinical depression, and a chronic sleep disorder. She diagnosed chronic tension headaches secondary to lumbar muscle spasms. In all other respects she found B, at least from a mental point of view, to be perfectly normal. She was very struck by the fact that B had almost doubled her body weight during the past eighteen months and that there was very little muscle in her limbs or over her back. The psychiatrist referred B to the pain clinic for pain management. She began treatment for anxiety and depression. Her husband and son had several joint therapy sessions with a family counselor. These enabled them to participate more effectively in the recovery program outlined for B at the pain clinic. The aim of her pain management plan was to help her take charge of her pain. The emphasis was on educating B about her pain, providing dietary and nutritional monitoring and a progressive mobilization and exercise program, and using TENS therapy to give her ongoing relief from the acute bouts of pain that continued during her recovery which took just over six months. Essential features of this approach were that each small step was explained and realistic goals were set. She was shown how to approach task management through organizing them into manageable bits. She was also shown effective techniques for stress management using her stress to her advantage rather than allowing it to weigh her down further. Within a relatively short time this help enabled her to take charge of her life though she continued to experience some manageable discomfort.

If you suffer from chronic pain, there are many aspects you will recognise in the story of B. The bottom line is *do not let your pain run your life*. You can beat it if you truly want to. You can do this with some help, but you must take charge to succeed. As a doctor helping patients with pain, I can only show them the way to recovery and provide relief along the way. It is the patient who must go for it.

CHAPTER EIGHT

Pain Management versus Pain Relief

Most people who have pain simply want to be rid of it or, at the very least, make it tolerable. What they seek is pain relief which usually involves taking medication, having injections, or even surgery. But sometimes these pain relief measures fail and the patient continues to have pain. The aim of pain management is to improve the quality of life for patients using approaches that help the patient cope and regain a productive and active life of which pain is a part.

When I discuss with patients these two different ways of dealing with pain – "pain relief" versus "pain management" – it is seldom simply a question of choosing one over the other. Patients often remark when a "pain management" approach has been recommended for them , "So there's nothing that can be done. I'll just have to live with it I suppose". This attitude of resignation and pessimism is not surprising because nearly every patient with ongoing pain has traveled a road of despair and experienced repeated disappointments when the relief hoped for was not forthcoming. Yet most patients do keep on trying to find relief at almost any cost. Life becomes a constant search for the Holy Grail of pain relief, "the perfect anodyne" (anything that relieves pain). There are techniques that, if properly used, will completely remove pain temporarily for almost everyone. It is sometimes beneficial to provide short-term relief (with injections of local anesthetic and steroid for example) to allow other treatment a better chance to succeed. But these temporary measures, even when repeated often, are not the solution when pain is a long-term or chronic problem.

The essential feature about pain management is that it requires the active participation of the patient, whereas pain relief requires only a passive role. You would think that most people would prefer to actively direct their care, but this is not so. The normal behavior of patients is to hand their problems to the doctor to solve. After all, isn't that what doctors are supposed to do; find the cause of what ails you and make the required decisions about treatment? This passive response by patients is at odds with our natural tendency to cling ferociously to our rights of self-determination in all other matters of importance. Most patients are hesitant, or sometimes even quite unwilling, to accept responsibility for their health or to initiate control of their pain. Encouraging patients to be in control is a major part of any pain management plan.

Pain clinics and services that use *pain relief* techniques are now increasingly available for the treatment of acute pain, such as that experienced after surgery. In contrast, *pain management* clinics are still not easily accessible for most patients because of the considerable demands on time and resources and the level of training required to staff them. There are distinct differences in approach and objectives in these two types of pain clinic.

Pain Relief Clinic	Pain Management Clinic
• doctor-directed care	• patient-directed care
• treat physical symptoms	• promote health/mobility
• use drugs, injections, and surgery	• use stress management and relaxation
• short-term relief aids recovery and mobility	• promotes long-term change of lifestyle and attitude
• minimize disability	• control and cope

Some clinics, such as that at McMaster University Medical Centre in Hamilton, offer both relief and management programs and are staffed by a team of experts who have the skills to deal with all types of pain and their related problems.

The concept of a multidisciplinary approach to pain management was developed about thirty years ago by an eminent anesthesiologist, Dr. John Bonica in Seattle, Washington. Himself the victim of chronic pain, Dr. Bonica recognized that successful pain management meant providing comprehensive care of the person including his physical, emotional, and social needs. Despite the obvious benefits of this approach, there are still relatively few centers that have adopted it. Another important factor is that training of doctors in the field of pain remains inadequate. On a current worldwide scale, the great majority of doctors graduate having had little or no training or instruction on effective methods of pain management. The trend to more and more specialization only further compounds the problem of where doctors receive their knowledge about pain. For example, orthopedic surgeons train would-be orthopedic surgeons whose focus is on bones and joints, while psychiatrists train would-be psychiatrists whose interest is in emotions and mental disorders. Every doctor knows that pain is a multifaceted sensory, physical, and emotional experience yet their training leaves them ill-equipped to deal with it. Bringing together a group of specialists in the multidisciplinary clinic goes a long way toward solving this problem.

In parallel to the growth of reputable pain clinics there has been, unfortunately for many patients, a growth in the number of physicians and nonmedical personnel operating what are advertised as "pain clinics"; the staff are often not trained and use a "fringe treatment" approach. If you suffer from pain, in particular from chronic pain, the last thing you need is another dose of ineffective medicine. Your family doctor will be able to refer you to the nearest pain clinic staffed by experts who are experienced in dealing with your type of problem. Ask about your pain doctor's qualifications which should include extensive training in pain management and a specialist certificate.

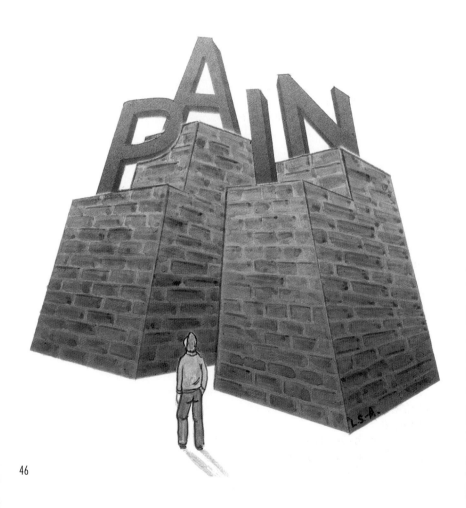

How to Manage Your Pain

Your pain is unique to you and a pain management plan must be worked out for you alone to satisfy your specific needs and abilities. There are some general principles that can be used by everyone, but only you will know if the details of a pain management plan will work for you. Your confidence of success must be reasonably high even though, at the beginning, you may have some doubts. In working out your pain management plan with your doctor you need to have a good idea of the goals most important for you to reach. These goals will then be separated into smaller, more manageable ones to form part of your plan.

The major goals of any pain management plan are:

- understanding your pain
- controlling your pain
- achieving wellness

Understanding Your Pain

You must know what your pain is (a very unpleasant sensory and emotional experience) and what it is not (something for which nothing can be done). Knowing your pain means knowing the boundaries or limits of your pain as much as knowing what it is all about. Imagine your pain was taken from you and pressed out flat so you could see the whole picture of your pain. It would then be quite easy to understand what it is and what peculiar features it has that need to be erased or changed.

If you have chronic pain (the worst kind), you probably have convinced yourself that nothing can be done to ease it. By getting to *know* your pain instead of

47

just *feeling* it, you will be able to map out the way to control it.

We tend to think of pain in terms of injury. Even the international definition of pain is in the context of injury.

Acute Pain

All acute pains are closely related to injury to the tissues, either actual, such as with surgery or trauma, or potential, such as with certain types of biochemical change. Acute pain alerts you that something has gone wrong in your body. It prompts you to take action, to instantly withdraw from the external cause of your pain (e.g., a hot flame), or to seek help from your doctor. We all think acute pain will probably be temporary and that it can be fixed. In other words, if you have acute pain you have no serious doubts that you will get better as the injury heals. *There is a purpose to acute pain*: it warns us of danger, and it is something that we can understand.

Chronic Pain

Most chronic pains begin acutely and progress to the chronic stage because they have not been relieved earlier. If you have chronic pain, it is quite normal for you to believe the original injury is still present and that, if you do certain things like exercise, the injury will become much worse. In reality, the original injury nearly always heals fairly quickly, but the feeling of insecurity and fear of worsening pain usually prevent you from doing the very things that would help improve your pain. *Chronic pain serves no useful purpose* and to date we have no adequate explanation of why some of us have it. Sometimes chronic pain is associated with an ongoing pathological process, (e.g., arthritis), but even in these cases pain can be felt in joints without any evidence of inflammation. Getting to know your pain is a bit like getting to know your big toe. If you wanted to get to know your big toe you would simply examine it objectively as if it belonged to somebody else. Your brain already has a picture of your big toe along with all other parts of your body, but it does not have a picture of your pain. You do not see your pain from an outsider's point of view because everything you feel about your pain is internalized. If you want to get to know your pain, you must first carefully examine all its facets, then gradually put the pieces together so that you have a clear picture in your own mind of what your pain is. Often patients have more than one pain, each with different features and felt perhaps in different places. To complicate matters further these different pains can be aggravated or eased quite independently.

Controlling Your Pain

The most important and most powerful force that can be used to control your pain is your own mind. Many people have learned to literally shut out their pain by using their powers of concentration, what we call "will-power". But there is much more to it than merely focusing your mind to eliminate your pain.

Clinical researchers often compare the effects of a real treatment, for example a pain-relieving drug, to that of a sham treatment with an inert substance that looks and tastes exactly like the real drug. They do this because one in three patients can respond positively when they receive *any* kind of "treatment". This is the *placebo response*. It is important to realize that these placebo responders are genuine and the effect is real. If they want to badly enough, people the world over can believe in the merits of whatever treatment is provided for them. The doctor's bedside manner is a powerful healing force when used properly, even when no real treatment is prescribed. It seems that for all of us, if the circumstances are correct, the power of the mind can be channeled to overcome physical ailments including pain.

My suggestion to a patient with chronic pain that this power of the mind can be harnessed to control his or her pain is usually met with a fair amount of disbelief or skepticism. Yet there are several effective training methods that enable patients to learn to control their pain using the power of the mind.

Biofeedback

This involves feeding biological signals from the body back to the patient, so that they can be manipulated at will. For example, your heartbeat can be displayed on a monitor and, with training, you can increase or decrease your heart rate as you wish. The heart beat is controlled by the autonomic nervous system. This happens automatically without our being aware of it; but the mind can override these automatic signals. In other words, your mind can take over willful or voluntary control of the part of the nervous system that normally functions unconsciously. By relaxing and concentrating on the task you can learn to lower your pain. For some patients this is a very effective method of pain control that can be applied whenever and wherever they wish.

Operant Conditioning

This method aims to change the behavior of patients who have pain. Often the predominant behavior in the pain patient is overly protective and tends to make the pain worse over a long period of time and delay recovery. In operant conditioning patients are trained to function differently for their benefit by rewarding desirable behavior (wellness behavior) and ignoring or punishing undesirable behavior (illness behavior). Attention seeking, inactivity, and inappropriate moaning and groaning may be undesirable behaviors depending on the circumstances. These actions, if ignored, would eventually cease. It is the aim of operant conditioning to actively discourage those behaviors in favor of alternative desirable behaviors such as being mobile. Operant conditioning is not the answer for everyone as it requires a high level of patient cooperation.

Hypnosis

For well over 100 years, hypnosis has been used to treat various mental and physical illnesses. Hypnosis involves placing the patient's mind in a trance, a state of mental dissociation lying between wakefulness and sleep. Instructions or suggestions from the hypnotist are used to alter behavior and thoughts after the patient is brought out of the trance. Repeated reinforcement of these instructions can produce long-lasting new behaviors and responses such as the lowering of pain levels. Some people can enter a self-induced hypnotic trance by using deep relaxation techniques. Although not everyone can be hypnotized, almost everyone can learn the benefits of relaxation.

Yoga

At one time, Western medicine opposed the idea that yoga might have significant health benefits, including pain control. Subsequently, many clinical studies have shown that yoga can aid wound healing and reduce stress-induced illness. As many types of chronic pain are aggravated by stress, yoga has become an accepted treatment for chronic pain. However, the body positions used in yoga are sometimes difficult for patients with chronic pain to assume because their joints are usually stiff from lack of use. The most widely used method is "hatha" which features a warm-up period followed by the taking of various positions and ending with deep relaxation and breathing. There are five basic positions that most people who are not overweight should be able to adopt:
- The *shoulder stand* which tones up the whole body, especially the spine, and eases back tension
- The *cobra* which eases lower back strain
- The *tree* which tones the leg muscles and relieves stress
- The *forward bend* which eases back strain and is said to invigorate internal organs
- The *half-spinal twist* which relieves tension in the shoulders, arms, back and neck

There is a form of Japanese yoga (*okido*) which uses repetitive movements and is especially suitable for anyone who is overweight.

CHAPTER TEN

Exercising Your Way Out of Pain

The three most important things about a successful pain management plan are *EXERCISE, EXERCISE, EXERCISE.* If you accept that fact, you are already on your way to recovery. Today, it is quite usual for patients to be up and walking around within a few hours after even major surgery because their pain is well controlled. Exercise is extremely important for recovery from surgery as a way of regaining muscle strength weakened by the stress of the operation. Recovery from surgery and recovery from chronic pain are really about achieving an adequate level of fitness. The word "fitness" is used to indicate the level of physical activity and endurance appropriate for your circumstances. On the first day after surgery your level of fitness will be quite low and you will only be able to take a short walk, slowly, and with assistance. As the days go by, your performance will improve and you will cease to tire so easily. You will finally reach a plateau of activity and fitness close to the level you had before surgery. This may happen in a week or so, but it may take much longer. At this stage you will have recovered.

Consider chronic pain in the same way. At the beginning of your pain management plan, your level of fitness is almost certainly the lowest it has ever been and you have probably gained weight. You promised yourself you would diet but somehow you could not muster the energy; besides, you tell yourself and anyone who listens, you eat hardly anything at all. The effort of getting started is too much, and so you slip into a shell of excuses and inactivity.

Begin exercising slowly. There is no short-cut to fitness. Your progress is going to be slow, just as it would be after major surgery, so try not to be in such a hurry to give up. Above all, *do not be afraid to keep moving even if you have pain.* If you have chronic pain you will not damage yourself with steady, graduated exercise; but you should realize that because of your long period of inactivity your muscles are going to be weak and easily strained. If you exercise too strenuously before you have achieved the required level of fitness strains will result, causing more pain, and you will probably give up once more. Remember when you were young, forever on the go, running until you were ready to drop, and afterwards how stiff and sore your muscles were? That is aerobic exercise. It requires you to be very fit. The exercises in your pain management plan are more gentle, progressive, and specific to certain groups of muscles involved in your pain. Training towards fitness ensures that you will become more mobile and increase your muscle strength.

The four most important activities for you to be able to do in your pain management plan are:

• sitting • lying down • walking • standing

We spend a great deal of our everyday lives doing these four things and if you have pain and are unable to do them, you are excluded from normal living. This isolation will make you feel more incapacitated by your pain and thoroughly miserable. At the beginning, your exercise program must be directed at enabling you to sit, lie down, walk, and stand without too much pain.

For many patients this first stage takes quite a long time – from two to six months. The second stage involves exercising more strenuously to increase overall fitness and to continue increasing the mobility of your joints. The last stage is a lifelong change in your daily habits to ensure that you will remain fit and active.

The key to exercising your way out of pain is to take it one day at a time, setting realistic goals that you can achieve. The exercises described here will get you started. Use the levels recommended at the beginning and work up from there.

Sitting Posture
Poor posture and poorly designed chairs are facts of life for many patients with back and leg pain. Tilting the pelvis backwards tends to flatten the lower back. If you already suffer from severe back pain this will make your pain worse, causing aches. It is important to use seating

that maintains the lumbar curve. A small cushion placed at your lower back will do. Your hips must be supported from the sides and the height of the seat should be such that your feet rest on the floor while your knees are supported. Measure the distance from behind your knee to the floor when you are standing. That is the ideal height for your chair. Your pelvis should be in a neutral position for you to be comfortable. Getting into or out of a seat is sometimes difficult if you have pain. Use your legs *and* arms to ease yourself into the seat and raise yourself from it. If you spend much of your day sitting, it is a good idea to get up, stretch, and move about every now and then.

Sitting Exercises

Sitting exercises will help correct poor posture and avoid muscle strain and tension.

Exercise 1: *The Tummy Tuck* Settle yourself into the seat and pull your body up as high as you can almost raising yourself out of the seat. Lean back then arch forward slightly and breath in deeply, holding your breath for five seconds. Exhale slowly and relax. Repeat this three times. This will tone up abdominal muscles and relax back muscles.

Exercise 2: *The Neck Roll* Sit up straight and look up at the ceiling. Breath in deeply and hold for five seconds. Exhale slowly and bring your head down slowly. Repeat, but this time move your head to your left side trying to touch your shoulder with your ear. Do the same to the right side. Repeat the sequence three times. This exercise loosens neck muscles and relieves tension.

Exercise 3: *The Pointer* Sit up straight in your seat, lift your left arm straight in front of you and point your index finger. Take a deep slow breath in, hold for five seconds, then exhale slowly. Repeat using your right arm. Do this sequence five times. Next, extend both arms and rotate your hands as if you are turning a door knob. Repeat the sequence three times. This strengthens arm and shoulder muscles and loosens the shoulder, elbow, and wrist joints.

Exercise 4: *The Toe Tap* Sit in an upright position with your feet pressed firmly on the floor. Take a deep breath and hold for five seconds at the same time as you lift your right toe off the floor keeping your heel firmly in place (as if you were going to tap your foot). Repeat with your left toe trying each time to lift your toe higher. Repeat the sequence five times. This loosens the lower leg and ankle muscles relieving foot strain.

When you are able to do exercise 4 comfortably, try this more strenuous exercise: sit upright, pushing your tummy forwards. Inhale deeply and lift your left foot off the floor, raising your knee above the seat, hold for five seconds, then exhale slowly and lower your leg. Rest for ten seconds then repeat on the right side. Repeat the sequence five times. This strengthens the quadriceps muscles on the front of the thighs and loosens the hip joints.

Your goal with sitting is to be able to sit comfortably for progressively longer periods. At the beginning you can expect to have some increase in your pain, but this should settle down within a few days. The entire sitting exercise routine takes about five minutes. You should try to do it at least three times every day.

Lying Down Posture

Having a good neutral posture when you are lying down is essential for sleeping and awakening refreshed. Your lying down posture is every bit as important as your standing or sitting posture. The three lying down postures are supine, prone, and lateral. The supine posture (flat on your back) requires a small pillow behind your head and a large pillow under your knees so your legs are bent. This tilts your lumbar spine into a neutral forward curve (lordosis). The prone posture (face down) should be used only with one leg drawn up, flexing the hip and resting your leg on a firm pillow. The lateral (side) posture requires a firm pillow beneath the head and a second large pillow tucked between the knees. Both the lateral and prone postures prevent back swaying movement during sleep that can cause stiffness.

Lying Down Exercises
There are two kinds of lying down exercises: stretching exercises and strengthening exercises. They are completed in sequence as given. Most lying down exercises should be done in the supine position.

Exercise 1: *The Foot Stretch* Stretching of the foot, ankle, and calf is done by rotating the ankle slowly one way then the other, a total of five times in each direction. Stretch your toes down slowly then stretch them up slowly. Repeat five times.

Lying Down Exercise 2: *The Pelvic Tilt* Tilt your pelvis backwards by pushing your back into the floor or bed. Inhale deeply and hold the position for five seconds then exhale slowly relaxing your back. Repeat five times. This is excellent for lower back pain and can be done frequently during the day.

Exercise 3: *The Hip Stretch* While lying on the floor or bed, clasp both your hands behind your left knee. Pull your knee slowly toward your chest, breathing slowly and deeply as you pull. Try to keep your back pushed into the floor or bed. Hold this position for five seconds and then relax. Repeat using your right knee. Repeat the sequence five times. When you are able to do exercise 3 comfortably try a double knee stretch (hands clasped behind both knees at once). This stretches both sides of your back at the same time.

Exercise 4: *The Lumbar Extension* This is done in the full prone position – face down, legs straight, and palms flat on the floor next to your head. Press down with your hands, raising your shoulders slightly off the floor, and inhale deeply holding your breath for three seconds, then relax. Repeat five times. When you are able to do this exercise comfortably, gradually increase the distance you push your shoulders off the floor, until you are able to push all the way up, so that your arms are straight. Let your stomach relax while you are in this fully extended position and let your back sag. Do not try to push your stomach to the floor. Hold for five seconds, then relax.

Hands and Knees Exercise

This is called the "hump and hollow" or "the cat". Kneel on your hands and knees, take a deep breath in, let your abdomen sag making a hollow of your back, and look up to the ceiling. Hold this position for five seconds. Relax. Breathe in deeply and arch your back upwards tucking your head into your chest and hold for five seconds. Relax. Repeat the sequence five times.

Walking Exercises

The importance of walking as part of your pain management plan cannot be stressed enough. If you are able to walk (you are not an amputee or paralyzed), this simple activity will loosen your pain. Some patients find they get the best relief from back and leg pain by walking briskly. Walking strengthens your leg and back muscles and improves your circulation. Also, walking takes you out and about, meeting people and generally enjoying life. The key to success in using walking as your primary exercise is that it should be interesting. Walking around a track or on a treadmill may be an excellent way to gain fitness and control your pain, but it will quickly become boring and you will lose your motivation to continue. When walking out of doors choose an interesting route. If you must stay indoors, walk while you are doing something else that is enjoyable like listening to your favorite music or reading.

Remember that the best walking exercise is done at speed. Better to walk a short distance quickly than to amble farther slowly.

Most patients who exercise, play sports or walk regularly before they develop pain, stop when pain strikes. This in itself can produce a withdrawal syndrome. Exercise, especially strenuous exercise, causes the brain to produce endorphins which give you a "high" and also increase your pain threshold. The result is that when you have pain, exercising vigorously makes you feel better and reduces your pain. The problem is that muscles quickly become weaker if you do not continue exercising. The earlier you begin exercising the better, and walking is probably the best way to start; but take things slowly and gradually increase the amount of walking.

For example: you suffer from chronic low back pain that sometimes radiates into your legs (sciatica) and makes it difficult for you to walk more than 200 meters before you have to stop and rest. This is a fairly marked level of impairment. Your pain management plan for walking should begin with your walking no more than 100 meters (out and back). Time yourself. The next day try to walk the same distance but a little faster. When you can do this distance as fast as you can walk with ease, set your target at 200 meters and go through the same routine until you are able to get out and back quickly and comfortably. Gradually from then on *your goals are to walk farther and faster* until you are able to walk as far as you want. For otherwise healthy patients the eventual target should be to walk at least five kilometers every day in less than one hour. But do remember that it may take weeks or even months for you to achieve this goal.

Begin walking on level ground until you can go at least a couple of kilometers with ease. Then try increasing the gradient using the same approach as setting your distance and speed goals. Rough ground may be especially difficult in the beginning because you need to constantly correct your body position but it is actually an excellent terrain to exercise on when your general fitness level is adequate. Once you are able to walk as far as you want, you should walk systematically for sheer pleasure. Wearing the correct shoes is essential if you want to walk in comfort. They should fit snugly and have a fully cushioned sole and a flat heel. They should be made of a lightweight material. Try to avoid walking in malls or shopping centers because concrete or marble surfaces are very hard on your knee and hip joints and your lower back. Having the correct walking shoes will enable you to survive these hard surfaces. If you work in a place with this type of floor, wearing these same shoes will help keep your leg and back pains to a minimum. Many patients (and doctors) who must spend long hours standing on a hard surface wear only footwear specifically designed to maximize comfort.

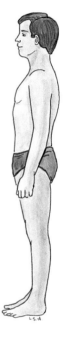

Standing Posture

Good standing posture is important for most types of acute and chronic pain. Pains over the back, neck, legs, and feet are affected by the way you stand. The general idea is to adopt a neutral position, as far as your back is concerned, and not to stand in one position too long as this aggravates strain. If you have been in the same position for a time and your back is aching, crouch down, or bend forward then back, stretching your back muscles. A good simple aid is a block of wood placed on the floor for you to rest one foot on. This tilts your pelvis and puts your lumbar spine into the most neutral position. You can achieve the same thing by putting one foot on top of the other.

Standing Exercises

Exercise 1: *The High Step*   Stand up straight with your feet apart (about shoulder width). Lift your left knee toward your chest (hold on to something for support if necessary), then lower it slowly. Repeat with your right knee. Repeat this sequence five times.

Exercise 2: *The Side Bend*   Stand straight with your feet apart and hands by your sides. Slide your right hand down the outside of your right thigh to your knee then back up to the upright

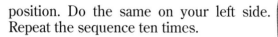

position. Do the same on your left side. Repeat the sequence ten times.

Exercise 3: *The Wall Slide*   Find a clear wall space where you can stand with your back to the wall and your feet together a little way out from the wall. You should feel your back pressing into the wall. Place your palms against the wall. Inhale deeply, and hold your breath for five seconds as you slide down the wall until your hips are level with your knees. Return slowly to an upright position. Repeat five times. Now turn and face the wall. Place your palms flat against the wall at eyelevel with your feet away from the wall. You should feel your back arching. Push away from the wall until your arms are straight. Then lean forward to the starting position. Repeat five times.

Exercise 4: *The Step Up*   This exercise requires a step – a bottom stair indoors or a doorstep will do. First, put your left foot on the step, then your right. Then step down with your left foot, followed by your right. Repeat five times.

The "step up" is a very simple and effective exercise that can be used to build up general fitness. As with all of the exercises the targets mentioned are the initial ones. As your fitness improves you should be doing each of these exercises faster and more often. Try to spend about 20 minutes each morning and evening doing these exercises. Remember to limber up before you start and to have a relaxation period after you finish.

The most frequent comment my patients make about exercise is that it interferes with other things they are expected to do. Mothers and fathers looking after children, or with a job to go to, must make time available for themselves that is dedicated to exercise. If you give all your time to other things and neglect your exercise, your pain management plan will quickly falter.

CHAPTER ELEVEN

How to Find Relief from Your Pain

Pain relief is distinct from pain management as it uses various pain-relieving drugs or therapies to block the perception of pain. Pain sensations can be interrupted or modified at three levels: in the tissues where pain receptors are active; in the central nervous system where pain pathways are located; and in the brain where the conscious awareness of pain is felt.

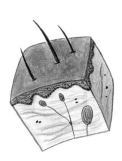
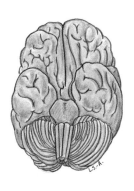

Using Drugs for Pain Relief

Several quite different classes of drugs are used to treat pain. The oldest and still the most widely used are *opioid drugs* or *narcotics* (e.g., morphine). Nonopioid drugs like the *nonsteroidal anti-inflammatory drugs* (NSAIDs) are extensively used for pain due to inflammation (e.g., arthritis), but are also used for postoperative and injury pain. Simple analgesics (e.g., *acetaminophen [paracetamol]*), are nonopioid, do not have anti-inflammatory properties and are used mostly for mild pain. *Local anaesthetic drugs* are used to freeze or block nerves that carry painful impulses and usually produce numbness. Other drugs commonly used as part of the drug treatment of pain include the *tricyclic antidepressants* (TCA), *sedatives,* and *receptor blockers.*

Opioid drugs

These are usually reserved for severe pains such as postoperative or cancer pain. However, some opioids are quite weak (e.g., codeine), while others are very powerful (e.g., sufentanil). Opioid drugs act in the central nervous system activating the descending inhibitory pathways to dampen the input of painful signals to the spinal cord.

The advantage of opioid drugs is that pain relief nearly always results when the correct dose is used. These drugs do not block pain, they only mask it. Quite often there is a feeling of being "drugged" that many patients find unpleasant. Other problems include a tendency to depress the control of breathing which can be dangerous in elderly patients and in babies. Constipation is also quite common, especially in the elderly, and can seriously weaken the patient. In young adults, the most common problems with opioid drugs are nausea and vomiting. All adverse effects of opioid drugs depend on the dose; the higher the dose the more likely they are to occur.

All of the opioid drugs share the potential for addiction or dependency. This can be *physical*, usual when these drugs are used to treat ongoing pain, or *emotional*. Fortunately, patients who have acute pain do not become addicted when given opioids. However, the opposite is true of those with chronic pain. Patients with chronic pain should not be given opioids if at all possible. The only exceptions are patients with chronic cancer pain who may require opioids as part of their palliative care. The World Health Organization recommends that opioids be avoided in treating mild to moderate pain, and suggest using a mild opioid for moderate to major pain and a strong opioid for severe pain. All patients should be given a NSAID or nonopioid as part of their pain relief plan, unless the use of this class of drug is contraindicated (in conflict with a pre-existing condition or treatment).

COMMON OPIOIDS USED FOR PAIN

OPIOID DERIVATIVE	MIXED EFFECT	SYNTHETIC
codeine	buprenorphine	alfentanil
diamorphine	butorphanol	anileridine
hydrocodone	levorphanol	fentanyl
hydromorphone	nalbuphine	sufentanil
meperidine (pethidine)	pentazocine	
morphine		
oxycodone		
oxymorphone		
propoxyphene		

Opioids can be given by mouth, injected intramuscularly or intravenously, given rectally as a suppository, sucked as a lollipop or applied as a skin patch. Some opioids are considered "weak" (e.g., codeine) but this drug is broken down in the body (metabolized) into morphine which is considered a "strong" opioid.

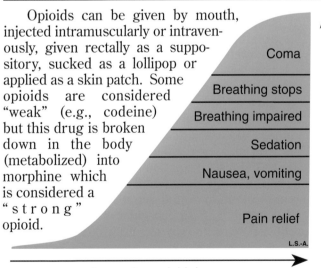

Coma

Breathing stops

Breathing impaired

Sedation

Nausea, vomiting

Pain relief

Increasing response

L.S.-A.

Increasing opioid dose

NSAIDs

These drugs used are most often for arthritis, postoperative pain, and pain from injury. They block arachidonic acid metabolism and production of prostaglandins which are the most important chemical mediators of injury and inflammation pain. They are

63

generally effective in controlling inflammation but not always in controlling pain. Pain relief is somewhat unpredictable with NSAIDs. For one patient one of these drugs might not work at all to relieve pain, while another patient may have very good relief. The newer NSAIDs seem to have a more specific action in blocking pain. For example, ketorolac is as strong as morphine in relieving pain. There are five different broad classes of NSAID though they all act basically in the same way. The oldest NSAID is aspirin and it is still the most widely used. NSAIDs are best suited for mild to moderate pain and are used with opioids for more severe pain. The advantages of combining a NSAID with an opioid are that the dose of opioid and risk of unwanted side-effects are reduced – *opioid sparing effect.*

NSAIDs can be safely used by most healthy patients. Some (ibuprofen, aspirin) are available over-the-counter. However, in some situations taking NSAIDs can be harmful. If you have poor kidney function, if you have a history of gastric or duodenal ulcers, if you have severe asthma or have a tendency to bleed easily, you should avoid taking NSAIDs. Also, as we get older, the function of our kidneys gradually deteriorates. Since almost all NSAID is excreted by the kidneys, we risk a steady accumulation of these drugs. There is thus a greater risk of serious complications such as gastric ulcers and bleeding and retention of potassium in the blood which causes the heart to beat irregularly. Because blood clotting slows down when we take NSAIDs, bruising and bleeding are more common. This could present a problem during plastic surgery or neurosurgery where bleeding may obscure the operation site and make it difficult for the surgeon to see what he is doing.

More than 20 different types of NSAIDs are currently available, most only by prescription from your doctor. We do not have enough information to decide if one NSAID relieves pain better than another. However, we do know that the risk of complications varies with the particular NSAID. Overall these risks are very small, from about 7 to 75 per million patients and mostly affect "at risk" groups of patients.

NSAIDs	
diclofenac	naproxen
fenoprofen	naproxen sodium
floctafenine	oxphenbutazone
flurbiprofen	phenylbutazone
ibuprofen	piroxicam
indomethacin	sulindac
ketoprofen	tenoxicam
ketorolac	tiaprofenic acid
mefenamic acid	tolmentin sodium

Other Nonopioids

The other nonopioid drugs are acetaminophen (paracetamol) and salicylates, (e.g., aspirin) which are only suitable for mild pain. Acetaminophen does not have anti-inflammatory properties but does bring down a fever and is therefore useful for many childhood illnesses. Aspirin should not be used by teenagers when they have a fever because it may cause a potentially fatal condition known as Reye's syndrome. Acetaminophen is often combined with other drugs like codeine which is a weak opioid drug. A common misconception is that these weak opioid plus nonopioid combinations are harmless. In fact, addiction to codeine is a major health problem around the world, especially in Canada, Denmark, and the United States which have the highest consumptions of codeine per capita in the world.

NONOPIOIDS	
acetaminophen	acetylsalicylic acid (ASA)
	aspirin
	choline magnesium trisalicylate
	diflunisal

Local Anaesthetic Drugs

These are the drugs that your dentist injects into your gums to "freeze" your teeth before he works on them. They block the movement of electrical pain signals along nerves preventing pain and producing

65

numbness. Once the local anesthetic drug wears off, movement of the signals resumes and normal feeling returns. Local anesthetics, in the form of injections, sprays and creams, are most useful when we need to block the pain pathways temporarily. The pain of childbirth is relieved by local anesthetics injected in the back to block the epidural or spinal nerves supplying the uterus and birth canal. Even the pain of having an injection can be prevented by using local anesthetic cream before the needle is inserted.

Local anesthetics rarely produce side-effects. Those which occur result from sensitivity to the drug or the administration of a very large dose which can cause convulsions or even death. The major differences between various local anesthetics is their duration of action and tendency to have side-effects.

LOCAL ANESTHETICS

chloroprocaine	articaine
procaine	bupivacaine
tetracaine	dibucaine
	lidocaine
	mepivacaine
	prilocaine

Local Anesthetics Combined with Steroids

Sometimes local anesthetics are injected together with steroids (natural substances produced by the body). For example, the removal of wisdom teeth often causes acute inflammation and swelling of the gums and is also very painful. Combining local anesthesia with a steroid such as methylprednisolone or betamethasone and injecting this before surgery greatly reduces these unwanted effects. Some types of acute back pain or large joint pain also respond well to injections of a steroid and a local anesthetic.

Trigger Point Injections

Many chronic musculoskeletal pains have pinpoint areas of very intense pain. These *trigger points* seem to be the source of painful stimuli causing more widespread pain within muscles and radiating to other parts of the body. The location of trigger points corresponds to acupuncture sites and it is thought that these may be active gates for pain signals. When active, trigger points become the major feature of the patient's pain symptoms. The "trigger point map" is useful because it pinpoints sites for the injection or spraying of local anesthetic to release the trigger which eases both muscle tension and pain. Sometimes inserting a needle, as with acupuncture, does the same thing. Massage therapy also can release trigger points and relieve tension and pain. Acupressure is a technique of vigorous rubbing and pressing at trigger point sites to relieve pain.

Counterirritant Drugs

The idea that irritation of an area of skin that is already painful will lessen the pain has led to the use of counterirritants. While it seems rather drastic to irritate an already painful site, it does appear to work. When capsaicin, an extract of hot chili peppers, is applied to skin, it blocks the action of substance P, one of the major pain mediators in damaged nerves. This blocks the pain. Some chronic areas of sensitivity, (e.g., after shingles) are also relieved by capsaicin, but its most useful role is in the treatment of pain from minor sprains and strains. There are no significant side-effects.

MOOD-ALTERING DRUGS

Many patients with pain require drugs that alter their mood and emotional reactions. Some of these drugs have pain-relieving properties separate from their ability to relieve depression and anxiety. The two broad groups are heterocyclic antidepressants and anxiolytics.

Heterocyclic Antidepressants

These drugs relieve depression. This is the main reason for their use. They also modify the actions of some brain chemicals, such as norepinephrine and serotonin, thus blocking the central parts of the pain pathway. There are therefore two reasons to use a heterocyclic antidepressant in patients with chronic pain – to relieve depression and to relieve pain. They also maximize pain relief from other drugs like morphine.

COMMON HETEROCYCLIC ANTIDEPRESSANT DRUGS			
amitriptyline	desipramine	imipramine	nortriptyline
clomipramine	doxepin	maprotiline	trimipramine

Problems associated with these drugs are common: mental clouding, slurring of speech, dryness in the mouth, weight gain, unsteadiness when walking, constipation, and difficulty in passing urine. Nightmares can occur which can sometimes be very disturbing.

Anxiolytics

This is a class of drug whose primary action is the relief of anxiety. It includes benzodiazepines, such as diazepam (Valium), lorazepam (Ativan), sertraline (Zoloft), and fluoxetine (Prozac). Sometimes these drugs *increase* pain levels because of where they act in the brain. It seems that anxiety can both lower and increase pain levels. When a drug like diazepam is used, it sometimes removes the factor that is actually holding the pain in check. Fluoxetine may alter your personality making it easier for you to cope with pain.

Sleeping Disorders

Disturbed sleep is common in patients with pain and leads to chronic fatigue and irritability. A number of drugs are used to help patients sleep, but almost all do not provide a natural sleep. When you take something to get to sleep, waking up is nearly always a problem. Amitriptyline, a tricyclic antidepressant, seems to be the best drug for normalizing the pattern of sleep, although even with it patients feel sluggish in the morning.

There is no doubt that taking drugs that alter your mood or your mind can be habit forming. This is especially a problem with benzodiazepines where long-term use can lead to a form of addiction. It is better to re-learn how to fall asleep restfully without the use of drugs. Occasionally it is necessary to use anxiolytics, for example, during periods of acute stress, but as a general rule you are far better off without them.

Patients often say that they will lie awake all night if

they do not have their "sleeping pill" but, almost any pill will suffice if they believe it will help them sleep. Relaxation is usually all that is required to get a restful sleep. But you should avoid late evening stimulants, such as caffeine in coffee, tea, or hot chocolate.

Receptor Drugs

There are numerous chemical mediators of pain receptors and pathways and some drugs have been developed that have highly specific, targeted actions. This class of drug has only recently been used for pain control but promises to be very useful in the future.

RECEPTOR DRUGS

Mediators	Blockers	Agonists	USE
serotonin	methysergide		migraine
	sumatriptan		migraine
noradrenaline		clonidine	menopausal flush
		dexmedi-	lower blood
		tomidine	pressure; pain
			control
NMDA	ketamine		anaesthetic;
			pain control
histamine	antihistamine		block allergic
			reactions, pain
prostaglandins	NSAIDs		anti-inflammatory
			pain control
bradykinin	NSAIDs (indirect)		anti-inflammatory
			pain control

Nondrug Approach to Pain Relief can be divided into those that stimulate nerves and those that interrupt nerve function.

TENS

Electrical nerve stimulation (TENS) is a technique of stimulating the large nerve fibers under the skin that send nonpain-related action potentials (electrical signals) to the spinal cord. This closes the gate to pain signals trying to enter the nervous system and relieves pain. Codetron TENS uses random stimulation and appears to be more effective than conventional TENS. The available TENS units are quite small and can be used daily while patients go about their normal activities. Clipped on a waistbelt or placed in a pocket the stimulator (about the size of a pack of playing cards) is connected by fine wires to a series of pads placed over the area to be stimulated.

Stimulator Implants

For some types of intractable pain, stimulation of the dorsal nerves requires placing wire electrodes close to the spine. Surgery is performed on the spine and the wire is brought under the skin to a radio receiver which is also implanted under the skin. A hand-held radio frequency generator beams a signal to the receiver stimulating the spinal nerves. A variant of this is a battery-operated radiostimulator which provides continuous stimulation. Implanted stimulators are suitable only for the few patients who are known to respond well. Electrodes placed at the thalamus, the main gate for pain in the brain, can also result in control of pain, but again this is not widely recommended because of the risks associated with brain surgery.

Summary

It is important to remember that pain relief measures are nearly always only temporary. Long term relief of pain depends on resolution of the causes for the pain. Resolution of acute pain follows recovery and healing of the wound or injury. In chronic pain, the causes are multifaceted. Rarely is chronic pain the result of persistent injury. It is most often due to maladaptation to the pain from the beginning. Recovery is a matter of restoring a sense of wellness and learning effective methods to control it.

The cancer patient is a special case. Pain relief and pain management are both equally necessary when the cancer patient has pain. In the chronic cancer patient who has no imminent threat to life, there is often an assumption that all or most of the pain is due to the cancer. This is incorrect. Most cancer patients require drug and other pain *relief* therapy, but there is no doubt that cancer patients also can have the same types of other pains that chronic pain patients have and these pains respond better to pain *management* methods.

CHAPTER TWELVE

Common Pain Problems

f you have moderate or severe pain, you should *always* consult your doctor for a correct diagnosis and appropriate treatment. It will not help you or your pain to delay because you do not want to bother the doctor.

For mild pain, you should use your discretion as to whether a visit to the doctor is necessary. You may simply need reassurance that you do not have a serious problem. Remember, pain is rarely very sudden *and* severe except for something like a heart attack. Most pain is mild as it begins and can then become more severe, sometimes very gradually, sometimes quite quickly. The earlier it is attended to the better. Once the problem has been identified, the approach used to conquer your pain will depend upon the choices offered to you.

The following descriptions of some common pain problems are given so you can understand better how different types of pain arise and what can be done about them. All pain benefits from the use of self-help methods of *pain management* which are often all that are required. Some pains, like surgery pain, often also require effective *pain relief* methods. It is a question of deciding what is best for you: relaxation versus a relaxant, exercise versus therapy, etc. Each person has a unique experience of their pain and while we can classify various pain states, relief measures depend on the needs and abilities of the patient.

Headache

Of all the pains that afflict us, headache can be the most distressing. Headache describes any kind of head pain – inside or outside the skull – and pains that radiate up from the neck. There are more than 100 different causes of headache. The most important categories relate to structures inside the skull (brain, blood vessels, membranes) or structures outside the skull (nerves, joints, muscles, skin) as well as sinuses, eyes, and ears. Headaches have several general causes:

- pressure on sensitive tissues
- pulling or distortion
- widespread dilation of brain blood vessels
- localized dilation of brain blood vessels
- prolonged muscle spasms
- inflammation
- painful nerves (neuralgia)
- disturbance of the central nervous system's control of pain
- hysteria (conversion) manifested as headache

Factors that can aggravate a headache are:

- movement of the head
- sensitivity to bright light (photophobia)
- sensitivity to loud noise (audiophobia)
- physical or emotional stress
- coughing, sneezing, or straining

Certain types of headache are caused by sensitivity of the brain centers to stimulant chemicals (e.g., caffeine). In some foods (e.g., cheese, especially cheddar) and in red wines, there are chemicals that are used by the body to manufacture the normal brain transmitters (serotonin and noradrenaline). When produced in large amounts these transmitters can cause migraine-like symptoms.

The headache from drinking too much alcohol (hangover) is essentially the result of the toxic effects of alcohol on the brain. Prolonged high intake can cause permanent injury to brain cells and severe mental illness. In chronic alcoholics headaches become less common as the brain deteriorates.

Although most of us have experienced headaches at some time in our lives, severe headaches are quite uncommon. Often headaches occur repeatedly over a period of years. It is very important to avoid taking drugs known to have the potential for addiction or abuse, unless they are absolutely necessary (e.g., during an acute and severe attack). Unfortunately many patients have become totally dependent on opioid drugs for the relief of headache when a simple analgesic or NSAID would be just as effective.

CLASSIC MIGRAINE Also known as "migraine with aura"
(due to dilation, then constriction, of blood vessels of the brain)

Features	Factors	Treatment
Preceded by aura	Familial (70%)	Prophylaxis
Most often unilateral	Abnormal stress responses	Stress management
Anorexia	Begins before age 20	Relaxation
Nausea and vomiting (early)	Foods (cheese)	Biofeedback
Photophobia	MSG, alcohol (red wine)	
Moderate to severe	Weather change	NSAIDs
Lasts 4-24 hrs		Ergotamine or DHE
Ratio of Female:Male, 2:1		Calcium channel blockers
		Beta blockers
		Tricyclic antidepressants
		Serotonin blockers

COMMON MIGRAINE Also known as "migraine without aura"
(due to pressure changes from brain vessel constriction)

Features	Factors	Treatment
No preceding aura		Relaxation
Mood disturbance	Stress related	Ice packs
Depression or euphoria	Familial (more than 50%)	Biofeedback
Hunger	Menstruation	
Fatigue	Changes in weather	NSAIDs
Photophobia	Foods (cheese, chocolate)	Ergotamine or DHE
Nausea and vomiting (late)	Caffeine	Serotonin blocker (sumatriptan)
Ratio of Female:Male, 3:1		Analgesics
Lasts about 8 hrs		
Throbbing pain		

CLUSTER HEADACHE (unknown cause)

Features	Factors	Treatment
Unilateral	Injuries	Counterstimulation
Sweating, tearing	Infections (viral)	Oxygen
	Emotional crisis	
Bouts (clusters)	Usually begins at age 30	Lithium
Red eye	Smoking	Ergotamine or DHE
Ratio of Female:Male, 1:4	Alcohol	Steroid prophylaxis
	Food (cheese, chocolate)	Calcium channel blocker
Lasts less than 1 hr	MSG	Serotonin blockers

MUSCLE CONTRACTION HEADACHES Also known as "tension or psychogenic headache" (due to muscle spasms)

Features	Factors	Treatment
Tight banding	Stress induced	Stress management
Occipital (back of head)	Muscle irritation	Relaxation
Photophobia uncommon	Muscle contraction	Biofeedback
No aura	Any age	Behavior modification
Aching neck muscles	Depression	TENS, acupuncture
Unilateral and bilateral	Caffeine	
Mild to moderate pain	Familial	Aspirin
Lasts 2-72 hrs		Acetaminophen
		Tricyclic antidepressant

WHIPLASH SYNDROME Also known as "acceleration-deceleration injury" (mostly due to automobile accidents)

Features	Factors	Treatment
Delayed pain (12-24 hrs)	Hyperextension injury	Cervical support (less than 8 wks)
Neck pain+stiffness (100%)	Stress responses	Neck exercise
Headaches (67%)	Anxiety	Heat/ice
Shoulder pain (33%)	Depression	TENS
Upper back pain (33%)		
Arm and hand pain (10%)		Analgesics
		Muscle relaxants
		NSAIDs
		Local anesthetic injections
		Steroid injections

Neck Pains

Pains in, and arising from, neck structures are common. The neck is one of most complex anatomical areas of the body and is densely packed with sensitive tissue. When you consider that an adult skull weighs more than 2 kilograms and is entirely supported by the neck muscles, ligaments, and bones of the upper spine, it is no wonder that pains often occur there.

MYOFASCIAL NECK PAIN SYNDROME
(due to acute or chronic muscle strain, spasms)

Features	Factors	Treatment
Trigger points over neck	Injury	Trigger point release
Trigger points over	Strains and	Injection therapy
shoulders	spasms	Relaxation
Muscle spasms	Damp weather	Biofeedback
Depression	Strenuous	Stretch exercise
	exercise	
Fatigue		Antidepressants
Nausea		NSAIDs
Constipation		Analgesics
		Muscle relaxants

Back Pains

Back pains are most common in the lower back (lumbar) because it is there that the upper body is supported. When we bend forward, tremendous stresses are focused on the lower back. If you have ever tried to lift a broom by the end of the handle, you know that great force is required. The same is true if we bend over to pick up something heavy. The marked additional leverage needed causes lumbar muscles to be stretched to their limit. More than 90 percent of all lower back pains are due to simple strains that recover within a few days or weeks. Often pain is not limited to the back but radiates into the flank or buttocks or even down the legs (sciatica).

The structures that can be involved in back pain are muscles, facet joints (a double set at each of the 24 vertebrae: seven in the neck, 12 in the chest and five in the lumbar part of the back), ligaments, spinal nerves, and discs (pads between the vertebrae).

LOW BACK STRAIN Also known as "mechanical low back pain" (due to overstretch of muscles and ligaments)

Features	Factors	Treatment
Very common	Strain and injury	Brief period of rest (less than 7 days)
Central pain (lumbosacral)	Poor posture	Exercise, gradual stretch
Radiating pain (above knee)	Previous back pain	TENS, acupuncture
Anxiety	Obesity	
Aggravated by straining	Inactivity	NSAIDs
Muscle spasm	Depression	Muscle relaxants
Impaired movement	Facet joint disease	Tricyclic antidepressant
Ratio of Female:Male, 2:1		Analgesics

SCIATICA Also known as "neurogenic or discogenic pain" (most often referred pain, sometimes due to disc prolapse)

Features	Factors	Treatment
Aggravated by movement	Strain injury	Brief period rest (less than 7 days)
Pain radiating below knee	Nerve root irritation	Exercise (walking)
Leg pain worse than back pain		
Worse on sitting	May have disc prolapse	Relaxation
Rod-like pain	Obesity	TENS
Sometimes numbness		
Sometimes muscle wasting		
Muscle spasms, cramps		NSAIDs
Ratio of Female:Male, 1:1		Analgesics
		Local anesthetic injections
		Steroid injections
		Back surgery (rare)

Chest Pains

Chest pains are most often the result of acute disease of the heart, lungs, or esophagus (food tube to the stomach) but pains also arise in the chest wall, ribs, and intercostal nerves between the ribs. The clinical features of chest pains aid in the diagnosis of the underlying cause. Thus pain located at the front left side of the chest and extending into the neck suggests myocardial ischaemia (the forerunner of a heart attack). Pain during breathing and localized to one part of the chest suggests pleurisy (inflammation of the outer lining of the lungs). Lower front chest pain and a feeling of heaviness after a meal suggests inflammation in the lower esophagus from stomach acid. Pain in the chest is sometimes referred pain from diseased organs in the abdomen. Thus, gall bladder pain can radiate to the right shoulder, pancreas pain can radiate to the upper back, duodenal pain can radiate to the right chest, and pain from the spleen can radiate to the left shoulder. Essentially, chest pains may not all be what they seem. Perhaps the most devastating and distressing chest pain is that of shingles which is caused by the virus that also causes chicken pox.

SHINGLES
(due to herpes zoster viral infection)

Features	Factors	Treatment

Acute phase
  line of blisters
  radiating pain
  sensory nerves affected
	Depressed
	  immunity
	Usually elderly
	Coincidental
	  diseases
		Acute Phase:
		  antiviral drugs
		  steroids
		  tricyclic
		  antidepressants
		  vitamin B12 and
		  complex

Chronic phase
  healed blisters
  hypersensitivity to touch
  sharp radiating pain
  thoracic (50%)
  neck (10-20%)
  face (3-20%)
  crawling underskin
  (formication)
		Chronic Phase:
		  analgesics
		  tricyclic
		  antidepressants
		  capsaicin cream
		  local anesthetic
		  cream
		  nerve injections-
		  steroid
		TENS, acupuncture

Abdominal Pain
Like chest pain, abdominal pain most often is acute and the result of pathology of the abdominal organs.

These include the stomach and intestines; the liver and spleen; the pancreas; the kidneys; and various other structures, such as mesentery (suspends the gut), blood vessels, and the lining of the abdomen (peritoneum) which, if inflamed, causes peritonitis. Infections of an organ are described by using the prefix for the organ and adding "itis" e.g., gastritis (stomach), colitis (colon), pancreatitis (pancreas). Most abdominal pains are diffuse cramping pains. Some can be very severe such as acute colic (kidney, gallbladder, intestine, or uterus). Chronic abdominal pain is uncommon and due mainly to inflammatory bowel disease or pancreatitis.

ACUTE RENAL COLIC
(due to kidney stone impacted in ureter)

Features	Factors	Treatment
Sudden severe flank pain	Recurrent kidney stones	Analgesic injections
Radiates to the groin		Fluids
Nausea and vomiting		Spasmolytics
Spasm of ureter (tube between kidney and bladder)		

CHRONIC PANCREATITIS
(due to inflammation of the pancreas)

Features	Factors	Treatment
Midupper abdominal pain	Alcohol abuse	Analgesics
Radiates to back	Tumors	Nerve injections
Burning, deep pain		Celiac nerve obliteration
Periodic attacks		

Childbirth Pain – Pain without an Illness

Until the twentieth century, childbirth pain was viewed as necessary and efforts to alleviate it provoked the wrath of religious leaders who claimed that this was unnatural. Today, women expect to have a certain amount of pain during pregnancy and childbirth, but the availability of many different approaches to pain control makes pain from childbirth very much a matter of choice. During pregnancy, the growth of the baby adds extra weight and stresses the lower back. Sometimes excessive pain during pregnancy is a prelude to considerable pain during delivery. As birth approaches, hormone changes soften the ligaments that bind the pelvic bones together. Other joints – hips, knees, ankles, shoulders, and spinal joints – also become more supple. For women who suffer from arthritis, these changes bring welcome relief from joint pain. Early labor begins with weak contractions of the uterus and as labor progresses the contractions become stronger and more uncomfortable. The change from painless early contractions to painful forceful contractions is usually gradual, but is accelerated as the second stage of labor arrives and the baby's head emerges. It is important to distinguish between the force of uterine contractions (cramping pain) and the pressure on sensitive pelvic tissues (sharp pain) which also causes referred pain to the lower back. The words that women use to describe childbirth pain are: *sharp, cramping, aching, throbbing, stabbing, hot, shooting, tight,* and *heavy.* About half describe the experience as tiring and about 40 percent describe it as exhausting, presumably because of the physical effort expended over a relatively long period.

CHILDBIRTH
(due to contraction of uterus and stretching of pelvic tissues)

Features	Factors	Treatment
Associated with labor	Previous experience	Relaxation
Progressive intensity	Physical stature	TENS
Mostly ends with delivery	Training	
Postnatal cramps	Marked obesity	Inhaled nitrous oxide
Sharp, cramping, tiring	Culture	Analgesics
		Epidural local anaesthesia
		Epidural opioid
		Spinal (uncommon)
		Pelvic nerve block

Natural childbirth (without pain or fear), introduced by Dr. Grantly Dick Read more than 50 years ago, greatly improved the overall experience for mothers but many studies showed very little difference in actual pain intensity levels. What was and is different is that *trained* mothers have better control of their physical and emotional responses to pain. Modern drugs and techniques for pain relief during childbirth are safe and effective giving the mother a wide choice of how to deal with her pain. Except in very rare circumstances, it is no longer necessary to anesthetize a mother for Cesarean section or forceps delivery. The use of "awake techniques" with epidural analgesia allows mother-child bonding.

Fibromyalgia
This condition is characterized by general pains, multiple tender points (at least 11 of 18 designated points), fatigue, insomnia, and joint stiffness. Patients with fibromyalgia (painful muscles and ligaments) are most often women (the ratio of females to males is 10:1), in their childbearing years (more than 80 percent are 30 to 50 years old), whose pain is aggravated by changes in the weather, menstruation, stress, and physical activity. Irritable bowel and chronic headaches are common. Most patients with fibromyalgia have marked disability yet do not appear ill. Depression often further aggravates pain and feelings of hopelessness. Metabolic changes in the muscles make them weak and achy. Also, the levels of most of the chemicals involved in the pain pathways are elevated. One theory holds that fibromyalgia is caused by progressive development of muscle microinjury where the load on a muscle becomes greater than it can handle. This produces muscle weakness where even lower loads are no longer tolerated without pain. Yet another theory states that fibromyalgia is the result of abnormalities in the central nervous system. In the past most doctors believed this to be the case and treatment was essentially psychiatry-based. Today there is enough evidence of structural and functional changes in the muscles and pain chemistry to discount this theory. Most patients *do* have psychological effects but these are not primary; rather, they are responses to the severe pain experienced by

most fibromyalgia patients. Only one in four patients with fibromyalgia has a history of injury, but more than one-half have a family history of the condition.

FIBROMYALGIA Also known as fibrositis, muscular rheumatism, and myositis (unknown cause)		
Features	**Factors**	**Treatment**
Generalized pains (94%)	Stress	Exercise, fitness training
11 of 18 tender points	Changes in weather	Nutrition
Ratio of Female:Male, 10:1	Menstruation	TENS
Fatigue (85%)	Obesity	Biofeedback
Insomnia (62%)	Familial (more than 50%)	NSAIDs
Depression and anxiety	Injury (less than 25%)	Tricyclic antidepressants
Joint stiffness		Sympathetic blockers
		Analgesics
		Tender point injections

Arthritis

Inflammation in joints causes destruction of the joint surface (synovial lining) and produces chemical irritants, but does not always produce pain. There is generally a good correlation between pain and inability to move the joint normally, but there is little relation between the amount of pain and the amount of disease in joints. Many patients with x-ray and laboratory evidence of severe arthritis do not have marked pain, while other patients, with few pathological changes, experience a great deal of pain.

On the other hand crystal-induced arthritis (gout) relates directly to the damage in joints and surrounding tissues. Some types of arthritis are "wear and tear" such as osteoarthritis, while others, such as rheumatoid arthritis, are due to abnormal immune function.

Slightly more than half of all patients with arthritis say that it bothers them all the time, while nearly two-thirds say it bothers them a great deal. Sometimes the pain arises in the covering of the joint (capsule and bursae), from inflammation (capsulitis or bursitis), or in the ligaments attached to the joint (tendinitis). This type of pain is quite common and made worse by movement. It is also very sensitive to even light touch. It is usually caused by overuse or severe strain, but the joint itself is not involved and swelling is minimal, in contrast to arthritis where swelling is usual.

Mechanical instability can cause joints to dislocate. This can occur repeatedly and cause pain. The shoulder, with its shallow socket, is the most commonly dislocated joint. Patients who sleep on their sides are more likely to dislocate their shoulders if they have their arms stretched above their heads.

Chronic or repeated injury to a joint can cause new bone to form. This distorts the joint and results in pain. This type of pain is associated with impaired movement. It is rare for tumors to occur in joints and cause pain. More often, tumors spread to bones causing softening or fractures.

Most patients with pain from arthritis find their pain is much worse when the joints are stressed by movement (e.g., walking), by pressure (the weight effect of sitting), or by changes in the weather.

Surgery for arthritis is sometimes necessary to restore function. Today, insertion of a fine tube into the joint (arthroscope) permits the surgeon to operate without having to open the joint. This speeds recovery and avoids more major procedures.

RHEUMATOID ARTHRITIS
(due to immune factors)

Features	Factors	Treatment
Small and large joints		Light exercise
Joint pain and deformity++	Rheumatoid factor (85%)	NSAIDs
Progressive disability	Weather changes	Steroids
Ratio of Female:Male, 2:1	(not eased by rest)	Gold salts
Insomnia		
Fatigue		Joint replacement surgery
Joint stiffness		
Age 20 and up		

OSTEOARTHRITIS
(due to "wear and tear" degeneration)

Features	Factors	Treatment
Large more than small joints	Previous inflammation	Light exercise
Joint pain and deformity	Injury	NSAIDs
Joint stiffness	Obesity	Nutrition
Age 40 and up	Weight bearing (eased by rest)	Joint replacement/ fusion
		Tricyclic antidepressants
		TENS

Phantom Pain

This is the pain felt after loss of a limb or other part of the body. Your brain's picture of your leg or arm is imprinted in childhood. If you lose a leg traumatically or by surgery, your brain's image of the missing part remains firmly in place. If your leg was painful before or during amputation the pain will also be imprinted. There is now a painful image in your brain that causes great anguish. In most patients the phantom images gradually decrease by a process called telescoping. This sometimes distorts the image and leads to transference of pain to other areas of the body. Phantom pain can be extremely debilitating.

PHANTOM PAIN
(due to painful images in the brain)

Features	Factors	Treatment
Often very severe	Severe pain at amputation	Relaxation
Episodic	Stump complications	Behavioral modification
Sharp plus dull	Neurotic personality	TENS, acupuncture
Felt in missing limb		
Ratio of Males:Females, 3:1		Preemptive analgesia
Any age		Nerve blocks
Affects 5% of amputees		Analgesics
		Tricyclic antidepressants
		Sympathetic blockers

Cancer

More than 30 percent of cancer patients do not experience pain. The majority of their pain is the result of infiltration of bones or other tissues by the tumor. However, cancer patients also have the types of pain that others might experience. Thus headaches, muscle cramps, or joint stiffness in the cancer patient do not necessarily mean the cancer is involved. Having cancer is a great psychological trauma and most cancer patients have changes in mood that require therapy.

The causes of the aggravation of pain in the cancer patient are primary cancer therapy (surgery, chemotherapy, radiotherapy); diagnostic procedures (CT scan, MRI, myelogram); or procedures intended to relieve pain (nerve destruction). Cancer patients are five times more likely to have shingles and ten times more likely to have osteoporosis (softening of the bones).

The drug treatment of cancer pain uses the World Health Organization analgesic ladder:
- all patients are given NSAID
- those with mild pain are given NSAID only
- those with moderate pain receive NSAID plus a mild opioid such as codeine
- those with severe pain are given NSAID plus a strong opioid such as morphine

---

CANCER PAIN
(due to infiltration of body tissues or obstruction by tumor)

Features	Factors	Treatment
Deep aching pain	Depends on tumor type	Relaxation, psychosocial support
Episodic stabbing pain		Tumor therapy
70% have cancer pain		WHO analgesic ladder
Insomnia		Tricyclic antidepressant
Marked fatigue		Anticonvulsant drugs
		Nerve interruption

Surgery Pain

Before the introduction of anesthesia in 1840, surgery was accompanied by terrible pain despite the liberal use of narcotic drugs or alcohol. Even quite recently postoperative pain was accepted as "normal" if you had had surgery. We now know that if you have moderate or severe pain after surgery, you are more likely to have complications, take longer to recover, and remain longer in hospital. Recently, acute pain services have been organized in every major hospital to provide effective control of surgical pain and an opportunity for every patient to undergo surgery without significant discomfort. This is a large undertaking but, for patients and their caregivers, the effort is well worth it. Today, there is no reason for any patient – young, middle-aged or elderly – to be afflicted with pain after surgery unless resources for acute pain management are not yet available. The era of painless surgery and painless recovery has arrived.

One important development is the introduction of *patient controlled analgesia* (PCA). A pump, operated by the patient, delivers pain medication into a vein (intravenous), under the skin (subcutaneous), or to the membrane and nerves around the spine (epidural). The pump is set by the doctor or nurse using a programmable computer to deliver a small dose of medication when the patient presses a button. There is no possibility of an overdose as the pump is tamper-proof. By this system, the patient who needs pain medication can receive it immediately. No more delays while the nurse is called, checks out the medication, then comes back to deliver it. PCA also gives the patient the choice as to how much medication to take and when to give it. PCA is suitable for children and adults and is cost-effective in spite of the expense of the computer and pumps. Depending on the type of surgery, the need for analgesia will vary from medication by mouth such as an opioid or NSAID (after minor surgery); by intravenous or intramuscular injection, usually an opioid or injectable NSAID (after minor or major surgery); or epidural or spinal injection of an opioid or local anesthetic (after major surgery). Whatever the actual method used, it is almost guaranteed that pain after surgery will not occur.

SURGERY PAIN
(due to the surgical wound)

Features	Factors	Treatment
Sharp or dull pain	Type of surgery	
At site of surgery	Age	Analgesics
Hypersensitive	Psychological	PCA
Decreases with healing	Cultural	Opioids
Maximum pain 0-24 hrs	Prior drug history	NSAIDs
Causes weakness		Epidural opioids
Causes insomnia		Epidural local anesthetics
		Nerve blocks
		Sedatives

Summary

The IASP has classified all types of acute and chronic pains, syndromes, and associated conditions. There are more than 200 distinct pain syndromes, far too many to cover in this book. The types of pain selected here illustrate some of the features of pain and act as a general guide to the causes of pain and ways to find relief.

INDEX